To my Children

Medea
Neriah
Joshua

This book would not have been possible
without the three of you.
You helped me onto the right path.
I am extremely proud and grateful
to be your mother.
I love you.

TWENTYSIX – Der Self-Publishing-Verlag
a cooperation of Random House and BoD – Books on Demand

© 2017 Sabine Metzinger
Production and Publisher:
BoD – Books on Demand, Norderstedt

ISBN: 978-3-7407-2657-7
Illustration: Coverfoto © blobbotronic/Fotolia.com
Translation: Herb Quick with Gabriella Bertelmann and Thomas Schneider for QCopy. www.qcopy.com
Further Participants:
Gerhard Kilian, 77837 Lichtenau, Germany, Editor

Table of Content

Part 1

1. Success	7
2. Fear	17
3. From the Fear of Poverty to Wealth	25
4. From the Fear of Illness to Health	37
5. From the Fear of Death to Living	52
6. From the Fear of Loneliness to Love	63

Part 2

1. Longing and Desire	73
2. Trust	84
3. Inner Dialogue and Autosuggestion	93
4. Observation, Personal Experience and Knowledge	100
5. Intellect and Understanding	111
6. Fantasy and Imagination	121
7. Action	132
8. The Subconscious	148
9. Self-Awareness	162
10. Determination	168
11. Perseverance	177

12. The Power of Community	185
13. Union – A little different Meaning of Sexuality	195
Summary and Essence	214
THANKS	230

Sabine Metzinger

Fucking Perfect

Success and the Ethic of our Soul

PART 1

1. Success

I had a dream and it was unbelievably vivid. I dreamt that there is a paradise. In this dream, I sensed that this vision could somehow become true, and that this life is meant to be much easier. I dreamt that peace, health, prosperity and love could live within me and everywhere in this world. Under these circumstances, life would be a celebration. I experienced all of this, as if it were already real. When I awoke from the dream, I knew with every cell in my body, yes! This is possible! But how?

Nowadays we are often confronted with spiritual phrases like: "Everything is all right, right now" and so on.
But, how can this be true, when we realize the circumstances on earth, in our society or even in our own little environment? And what is "true" and "false" or "right" or "wrong" at all and where leads this way? "Right" seems not to be meant in the context of ethics itself. Obviously there is something wrong, when there exists so much evil. "Right" seems only to be based on the fact, that an action causes a reaction and that we simply have to harvest what we sow.

Fear sustainably influences always what we call success and this seems to have us lead to such a worldview, which we have to face meanwhile. Is there a way to change success with only one heightened perception and use it in another and better way?

So – I think yes. And I will describe how to shift.
Then, we would be able to change not only the meaning of success in a positive way, but also our worldview and the understanding of ourselves as well. This new expanded approach would enable us to align our thinking, feeling, speaking and acting towards peace, happiness and love. A potential growth and change would cause automatically this way. It looks very much like we as human beings are figuratively speaking stocked in a

filial imprinting phase of our true potentials and abilities. The lack of knowledge about these circumstances brings along this world we created altogether. So, we can stop blaming each other, because everybody seems to contribute this unconsciousness on its own way. Similar to a baby, we also would not blame its attempts of communication and interaction when its development of mother tongue and body coordination is not as good as you find it when you are grown and have finished school.

What is success

Success itself is based on certain characteristics, without the interplay of which it is likely difficult to be or to become what we call successful. The characteristics on which we base our success are: Longings and Desire, Trust, Inner Dialogue and Autosuggestion, Observation, Personal Experience and Knowledge Intellect and Understanding, Fantasy and Imagination, Action, The Subconscious, Awareness, Determination, Perseverance and the Power of Community. We will examine the word "success" very carefully in this book, and repeatedly looking at the parameters of the various perceptions of success from different viewpoints because "Success" – or "being successful" – as interpreted and experienced until now, has been the source of a great deal of hardship, struggle, misunderstanding and misfortune.

Strictly speaking, "SUCCESS-FUL" merely means that a desired aim or purpose has been accomplished. Every action is followed by a reaction, and the more often this action is taken, the more often the reaction takes place. Thus we are FULler of „that what follows", and „that what follows" is our SUCCESS. When we think, say or do certain things – or refrain from saying or doing certain things – frequently, a certain reaction or result will follow in a corresponding frequency. So the "full" in "successful" refers to the quantity of the particular "success", and not

to its quality. Saint Francis of Assisi coined a quote that points to this misunderstanding:
"Start by doing what's necessary; then do what's possible; and suddenly you are doing the impossible."

The significant first step here for holistic success has been forgotten until now, leading to fatal misconceptions. Standing in the conventional understanding of success, we already expect a certain desired quality – in other words, the second step – from the outset, without consciously evaluating the quality of the initial action beforehand. We are continuously trying to achieve the possible without paying attention to the necessary, all the time wondering why everything seems so impossible.

Our complete responsibility for ourselves and everything that is, lies hidden in this misconception. The "response" in responsibility points to the fact, that a fundamental truth about ourselves is at play here. What is this variable X, that we have forgotten to include in our equation of life? Maybe the true awareness about, who we really are?

It is not only love that multiplies when you share it, as sayings want to make us believe. That is not true. Everything multiplies if shared. Seen from a quantitative point of view, we are always successful, no matter what happens in our lives. No matter how horrible what we experience may be: it is always a result of the sum of our actions or acts of omission, and therefore our success. Everything that we experience is a consequence of our thoughts, words and actions. Initially, these consequences are entirely free from judgment; they are neither good nor bad, both on the large and small scale. Often, the impact of the own action or omission does not become clear – whether consciously or subconsciously – until some time has passed, so that our responsibility remains unrecognized.
Nonetheless, we have apparently always understood the laws of success. Our every molecule seems to be oriented towards

it, just as it is omnipresent in nature and our environment. Or has anyone ever heard of the necessity for a drop of water to go to school to learn, how to transform itself into steam under the influence of heat or the sun, so that it can defy gravity and rise to the sky, only to concentrate and condense? I am not aware of the need to teach a thus transformed drop of water how to become a drop of water again, or as a unique and perfectly shaped snowflake to fall back to the earth, in order to continue the eternal cycle of life. Why we human beings think that we don't operate according to the same laws that govern everything around us?

Actions and Reactions are Habits

According to the Merriam-Webster dictionary, habits are defined as *"a usual way of behaving; something that a person does often in a regular and repeated way"*, and *"an acquired mode of behavior, that has become nearly or completely involuntary"*.

Everything that exists today is based on the context inside of which we have defined and experienced success until now. Habits show the "how" of our relationship to everything that we ourselves are and everything that surrounds us. In other words, we only notice what we do, think, feel and say, when we begin to consciously pay attention to it.

Until now, actions and reactions (results) – that are not aligned with the values or wishes of ourselves or others, have been seen as failures. From the vantage point of our new and extremely basic definition of success, however, we can already surmise that we have been suffering under a fatal misconception.
What is failure really? In the German language failure is „miss-success". Interestingly enough, we have always defined failure as a lack of success, rather than a lack of quality or awareness

in the action and the reaction, as the original context of the German word would suggest. Instead of placing the focus on the lack of success, the word failure or „miss-success" actually contains the solution. When we focus on the cause rather than the effect, we can actually see that something is indeed missing – the quality as well as the purposefulness of the originating action.

The Basic Motivation for Habits

It appears that the habits of so-called unsuccessful people are largely negativity or deficiency-motivated, whereas the habits of so-called successful people, for the very most part, appear to be positivity-motivated – they are oriented toward and motivated by abundance. Nonetheless, a certain background motivation seems to be missing, when we get present to the current situation and observe the results in this world on the large and small scale.

Basically we can distinguish two primary motivations for human beings. First, there is that, which we call fear or deficiency, and secondly, there is what we refer to as love or abundance. Everything that we have defined as failure until now is actually success, as much so as everything that we have called success. Whether "success" or "failure" – both are reactions to an action, and therefore both are a success seen from the vantage point of natural laws or success principles.

How can it be then, that we have a world that looks the way it does?
Well, all of us have collectively thought, felt, said, done – or refrained from doing – those things that occurred to us as the right things to do (or not to do) based on our interpretation of success until now. Instead of success as we have defined it, however, these things have produced the „miss-success" or "failure" that we see today. That which the collective

consciousness - we should actually call it collective unconsciousness - has created is, what we experience as success and failure, resulting all too often in violence and/or injustice, especially against the more vulnerable among us. The statement "I have no success" is based on a misconception. We are lying to ourselves, because we have never really recognized the actual scope of our responsibility and with it our power.

"You can never solve a problem on the level on which it was created." – Albert Einstein

This quote hits the nail on the head. Our present interpretation of success creates the world that we experience right now, with all of its violence and the increasing number of atrocities and injustices. The variable X, along with a new definition of success based on that variable, can transform that very same world into the paradise, that has always been there.

Our negative habits began very early in our lives – in early childhood – and grow like a perennial plant in the sequence of annual cycles time and time again. The seed germinates, ripens, carries its own seeds and dies, only to have the new seeds germinate again with the next cultivation. Consider, though, that a plant made of seeds carries a multitude of new seeds. And so it is with our strongest habit: the habitual way we define and experience success.

But far too often, however, we treat our negative habits, concerning success, as if they were weeds, having forgotten that those weeds possess healing powers. Weeds are medicinal herbs. And they are trying to tell us, what isn't working about our definition of success. Like those weeds, our negative habits hold a gift for us – they want to bring us healing, yet we pluck them out without paying any attention to what they are trying to tell us or making intelligent use of them. If we examine the origin of these habits, they will show us the path to our true potential and to the aforementioned variable X, and we will have a much easier time of uncovering our faulty definitions and misinterpretations.

Our habits originated jointly and severally from our familiar interpretation of success. Similar to a puzzle, we have already completed the frame. Many pieces are already in place. But the more similar the colors and textures of multiple pieces become, the harder it becomes to find the correct piece. We have placed some of the right pieces in the wrong place. We have removed critical pieces from our puzzle and laid them to the side, believing that they belong to someone else's puzzle. No wonder, then, that our picture of ourselves becomes ever more removed from the picture it actually should be. Fundamentally, we are familiar with the overall picture. However, we are missing the conscious view and the understanding of where which piece belongs, and that those pieces lying to the side are actually the pieces missing from our own puzzle.

In order to make use of the true power of our habits, it is enormously important that we first recognize and understand the curse of our negative habits that originated out of deficiency and fear motivation. The sum of these habits brings about the worldview that we live in today. Our habits bestow upon us massive wealth and massive poverty at the same time, as well as the impending doom of the planet upon which we live.

Far-Reaching Consequences

The true magic of our habits is than the reversal of the curse of our negative habits, and yet it is so much more than that. It's about creating our future successes in the same way, that they were gifted us at birth, and consciously setting actions that make sense and create happiness, fulfillment and love far beyond our current definition of success. This particular shift seems to be especially urgent at this juncture in human history. Reversal is therefore not enough, for we would be turning a curse into a blessing, and a blessing into a curse, and would still be in a polarity. The true magic of our habits lies behind it. It contains the resolution of the greatest misconception this world has known.

Exponential Growth

Exponential growth, in other words a quantum leap for humanity, is possible, if we integrate the missing or forgotten variable X in all of our thoughts, speech and actions. If we comprehend the information in this book as what it truly is, change can come easily, because everything is ok, right here and now, and nothing is for naught – what exists now is "fucking perfect" (forgive the provocative expression), and we can then recognize and understand that.

The following context illustrates how this exponential growth in a positive direction is possible. It has been documented that a company needs four positive employees to compensate for one negative colleague. It is much the same with habits: figuratively speaking, it takes four positive habits to compensate one negative habit. Here, we're simply replacing our "outer employees" with our "inner employees", represented by our habits. In both cases, it is the amount of energy or life force connected with these people or habits, that is required to maintain a balance.

Negative habits are based on negative beliefs, which generally join to form larger belief systems that in turn support and feed one another. The smallest common denominator among the belief system we call life is, directly after the misconception "love", the resulting misconception "success".

If we could bring ourselves to new, positive beliefs and habits in this regard, potential growth in the desired direction will follow. A veritable explosion of wonderful concatenations and events will come to pass. The sum of our negative habits is replaced by positive habits. Simultaneously, the capacities of the four bound positive habits are set free, since they are no longer required to compensate for the conglomeration of negative habits. The consequence is obvious: the domino effect changes direction and activates a series of useful and positive chain reactions. What's more, these released energy reserves in turn ease the process of integrating more and more new positive habits. For one thing, we are much more motivated by the experience of success that feels like a quantum leap. For another, we actually have more energy available, which in turn makes it easier to detect, distinguish and replace negative patterns and traits. At the same time, we come into contact with potentialities – new positive habits - that we previously knew nothing about, although they may have lain dormant in us.

A positive cycle of exponential growth can arise and will pull us along inexorably, if we allow it to. A cycle, we are familiar with from negative, undesirable chain reactions, only reversed: a cycle of the desired, wished-for, positive kind. Lastly, this path is in spite of its simplicity and banality the greatest challenge of our lives and human history, since it forces us to question everything that we held as truth until now.

The Consequence of Exponential Growth

As a consequence, sooner or later we will not only be capable of creating life the way we want it, but also of uncovering our true purpose and destiny, as well as the ideal way to express it. All that already lies within us, waiting only to be discovered or better to be remembered. Just as a tree does not need to be told which tree it will become, and no plant must be told which plant it will become – we also know which talents we are meant to express. We ourselves decide, when this will come to pass.

We have believed that we must forget, or more accurately, deny ourselves, and have struggled to become "good" or "someone better". We now have the opportunity to remember this misconception. To put it in the words of my mentor, Eugen

Simon, (success coach, author and founder of Gedankendoping): *"It is time to forget, what we have forgotten to forget, and to remember, what we have forgotten to remember."*

Remembering is an act of „being aware", so fore, self-awareness or consciousness. I would actually like to use an invented word here, PRIMEMBER, to represent remembering who we truly are – reMEMBERing the original, PRImordial version of our self. The more human beings primember who they really are and why they are here, the more the true magic of our habits can show itself. This magic is capable of bringing about the sought-after transformation of this planet, which we until now have believed to be impossible.
It is time to remember who we really are, who we have always been and who we always will be: a part of the DIVINE WHOLE, the EVERYTHING-THAT-IS – without compromise and with every consequence.

We will begin by examining our deepest fears together, before we take a closer look at the basic structure of our behavior based on the aforementioned success characteristics. We will examine how, where and why a particular characteristic is already being applied on the basis of a misconception, and how it could be applied in service of our responsibility to ourselves, and with that in service of our responsibility to our entire environment.

Your subconscious is waiting for this. It is on the starting blocks and led you to this book – perhaps unconsciously, but certainly not indeterminately.

2. Fear

Fears are shadows and don't really exist. They are assessments and judgments that emanate originally from the perception of our environment and occur to us as an unalterable, menacing truth. Nevertheless, they are nothing more than pure interpretations. They have been picked up from the environment, our families and society, who just know only this way of success and world. We experienced the fears of everyone around us – parents, friends and a multitude of others – and adopted them as our own truths. That happens without reflection when we are children. Even when we are grown, we have a difficult time recognizing and overcoming these phantoms. Moreover, we continue to propagate them - and by the way completely unaware of what we're doing - further infecting the world with our frightening misconceptions. Every time we articulate a fear, we sow the seed of that fear in ourselves and others, so that it is continuously strengthened and adopted anew. This happens at times even without a spoken word: hesitant, fear-based actions and decisions, or even those often underestimated failures to act or decide, also create chain reactions in our environment, legitimizing and strengthening our fears.

Needless to say, most of us would never intentionally spread fear. On the contrary, these events usually happen without any conscious awareness, and are all too often grounded in those deadly "good intentions". In many cases, it is hidden behaviors that fuel fears. The result, however, is always the same: fear carves its path, becoming greater and more powerful on the way.

The Impact of Fear

Fear deprives our personality of its charm and steals our clarity. It weakens our concentration. It undermines our perseverance, and sucks every bit of motivation and will out of us, leaving an inner state behind that resembles a parched salt lake. Fear tends to close every door and, in fact, deplete our entire belief in anything positive. If we give it enough power, it can even rob us of our positive memories. It seems as though the love within us dies. Fear paralyzes reason, undermines self-confidence and strangles all spontaneity. Insecurity runs rampant. Inspiration becomes a foreign word and seems light years away. Emotions get suppressed. Constriction arises and our bodies seem to hunch and tense up, as if by some invisible force. Insomnia and restlessness, lethargy, misery and doubt are common consequences.

It is fear that drives us to inflict damage upon ourselves and our environment – both people and nature – on a daily basis. Fears are thoughts that determine and direct our actions, and therefore our daily routine and our entire lives. Fears are self-imposed energies and misconceptions, that make their way from our inner lives to the outside world, to draw our attention to something.

And that is exactly the core point: They want to show us up, that we at that point, misunderstand our connection with ourselves and all that is around us, as mirror of the holy devine.

Our Mindset

That is why our mindset – our attitude toward this great divine spirit – is so important. Everything that doesn't inspire us stands as a separating entity between us and the Great Spirit within us and around us. Everything that exists is imbued with this energy; is this energy; is life. It is condemning thoughts that act as separating entities here. Condemnation - in German „MISS-JUDGMENT"- in this context is the expression of lack consciousness from childhood, which we learned to adopt and apply. Lack consciousness in this context refers not to a lack of material things or other benefits. Rather, it refers to a lack of awareness of our true divine universal origin and the power associated with it. By contrast, being deeply connected with the divine spirit within us results in evaluation - in German „JUDGMENT". Appreciation is the expression of abundance consciousness, which bestows upon us a feeling of deep love and bliss.

Love is not something that we DO; rather, love is something that we ARE in the moment, when we do something out of heartfelt inspiration, profound connection and joy. Then we are able to recognize the "original part of divinity" in everybody and everything that surrounds us. In this state of mind, any adversity can be overcome. This is, however, exactly what has been so effectively trained out of us. Thus it is hardly a wonder, that many of us often feel like having no control of our lives. The reality is, however, that we have learned to exercise a false control over ourselves and therefore a false way of power, strength and authority.

It is fear, along with all of its perceived consequences, that leads us to believe in less than we truly are and carry within us. These fears are actually capable of robbing us of all purpose, even if we are living in apparent prosperity. For there is one thing that fears will never give us – namely that, which we all long for: true fulfillment.

Filled with Fear: We Create What We Fear

True fulfillment, a state where happiness and satisfaction are predominant, will not be experienced with a fearful mindset. It would not be accurate, however, to claim that a fearful person is not capable of experiencing a state of fulfillment. Strictly speaking, we are also fulfilled when we have a fearful mindset. The word "fear-ful" speaks for itself here. When we wallow in deep fear, we are actually fulfilled – full of everything that fear has to offer. As already mentioned, it's not only love that multiplies when shared. Why else would our world look like that nowadays? All other emotions as well as the so associated actions are grounded in that same multiplying factor. The major difference between a mindset of true fulfillment and a fearful mindset is the consequences. True fulfillment generates a state full of happiness and love. A fearful person, on the other hand, will experience the opposite – misfortune, "bad luck" and malaise. The statement that fear robs us of all imagination is not entirely accurate. On the contrary: fears actually create an enormous playground for imagination and thus are instrumental in the process of the horror scenarios, that arise from imagining the worst possible outcome of a threatening situation. sooner or later this is becoming reality in one form or another. It is uncomfortable enough for a single person to look at their "failures". When an entire collective nurtures a particular fear or even several fears, this collective will subconsciously do everything to ensure that the dreaded reality occurs, for this too is success.

The Fear of Loss

The fear of loss is the fear from which all other fears can be seen to originate. It shows us that we have lost contact with our true origin.
Loss is equivalent to lack or deficiency and first and foremost, loss means that something or someone is missing, without which we believe we cannot live or survive. Basically, the big misconception lives right here. What's missing is the awareness of the connection to our true selves, which many of us lost very early on, because it is so effectively trained out of us. Therefore, we are lacking something that we consider natural and essential for survival and living. This misconception is the root of all fear, and forms the basis for our assessment of ourselves and of our environment.
If we observe fears and name them differently, we will get aware of the smallest common denominator, which is necessary for a fundamental change and the solution becomes visible. We define fears negatively, i.e. the fear of poverty, the fear of death, the fear of illness, etc. Causally, however, what

we really fear is the loss of prosperity/wealth, life or health. If we could realize that, we would think, speak and do completely other things in order to create what we really want instead of what we don't want. We would suddenly be able to get aware of the whole paths which led us to illness, war and poverty - to separation - and would change them. This reversal alone should be enough to clearly demonstrate how game-changing a shift in focus can be. These fears cause and nourish each other, and take turns in regard to intensity. Whether it's the fear of death in wartime, the fear of poverty during economic and financial crises, or the fear of illness – especially after wars and catastrophes – fear rules the world. We live in a world in which fears run increasingly rampant, and for good reason. We will be examining several fears and reasons more closely in the following chapters, for finding this „good reason".

One grave example of fear, or the absence of fear, can be found in Napoleon Hill's book "Think and Grow Rich". An entire collective of people let go of their fear of something and achieved something extraordinary:
During the "flu" epidemic, that broke out during the world war, the mayor of New York City took drastic steps to check the damage, which people were doing themselves through their inherent fear. He called the newspapermen and said to them, "Gentlemen, I feel it necessary to ask you not to publish any scary headlines concerning the 'flu' epidemic. Unless you cooperate with me, we will have a situation which we cannot control." The newspapers quit publishing stories about the "flu", and within one month the epidemic had been successfully checked. So powerful is the absence of fear.

The Power of Fear and its Abuse

There are people who are familiar with the manipulability of people and masses of people through the instrument of fea and who use this knowledge to further their own power-political and monetary goals. They use this knowledge for their own capital gains – both material and ideal. This has happened countless times, bringing humanity to its knees even at the threshold of its full bloom. Even Albert Einstein's grandiose achievements were turned into a political power toy – the atomic bomb. Here once again we see the effects of our erroneous definition of success and the fear of loss that causes manipulations grounded in some version of misconstrued "good intentions". Based on the interpretation of life from the viewpoint of what these people may believe, this may make sense for serving to achieve success and prosperity. But nevertheless something went forgotten – something that Gottfried Keller once expressed so beautifully: *"Study people not to outwit and exploit them, but to awaken and mobilize the good in them."* The only thing that would ensure an adequate application of all our discoveries and current achievements toward mastering our challenges would be a return to the principle, illustrated in this Gottfried Keller quote. This return comes about automatically, when fears are uncovered and we find our way back to self-love and true self-awareness. At that point, using our resources for anything but positive causes are only possible under severe emotional suffering. Pointing out reversely, it becomes a necessity for the ethics of the soul to follow the golden thread of the divine universal origin of all of us, and everything that is.

Currently, humanity is once again standing at the threshold of its full bloom. Evolutions are happening at a breakneck pace. Meanwhile we are faced with a plethora of catastrophic scenarios – enormous monsters that wander like phantoms through the media, feeding our fears. Everyone that adopts and nurtures this fear will think, feel, speak and act accordingly, thus playing their part in allowing these sketched-out catastrophes to become reality. We should use the above mentioned example of the „flu epidemic" and use it for our medias. Regardless of whether we are for or against the catastrophes, the focal point and the nucleus of the entire phenomenon is the catastrophic scenario. The focus is on the so-called evil or bad, so that it is almost forced to take place.

As Albert Einstein put it: *"The world is not threatened because of the people who are evil, but because of the people who allow the evil."* Catastrophes can be prevented, if the fear of it disappears and in the place of the catastrophic scenario a desirable scenario exists, for which actions are taken.
Everything that exists now can be used in a positive and beneficial manner. Nothing is for naught in this world. Yet only a return to the divine in us will cause us to use the key to all of our achievements for good instead of for evil.
As Gandhi said: *"You must be the change that you wish to see in the world."* The more people that are in touch with their divine core, the more people will know how our achievements are to be used. They will have access to that knowledge simply because they are connected to the great entirety, and because together we can establish a single goal: a new world – our paradise.

Media Abstention: A Step Toward Self-Awareness

Anyone who struggles with fear and whose fears are exacerbated by the headlines and articles in the media could serve themselves to undergo at least four weeks of media abstention, to observe what happens.
It would make sense to use the time during this abstention to closely study yourself.
The more we shut off manipulations from the outside, the more aware we become of our inner being. This process is critical in order to learn when we want to apply something differently, and how we should go about it, whether we are targeting ourselves or our environment.

Doubt and Indecision as Guides

Along this path, indecision and doubt will be constant companions. They often begin sowing their seeds in the underground, fully undetected. They are masters at disguise and deception, and they repeatedly promote new fear, doubt and indecision wherever they go – unless we learn to recognize how they can be utilized to our benefit. In this way they are similar to soccer players that are not allowed to play in their actual position. The team will only be successful when these players are placed in a lineup that matches their talent level.

Applied to doubt and indecision, this context means that if we apply these characteristics to our own benefit, they can decide the game for us, and show us, where the cause of our fear comes from and which treasure lay forgotten there. The more we do so, the more self-confidence we develop. As self-confidence grows, fear, doubt and indecision begin to disappear automatically. In this book you will find many examples of how we can use doubt and indecision to our advantage in order to transform our old "success world view" into a new one.

We are not aware that behind habits that we consider positive, is all to often fear as well. When we discover the misunderstandings of these fears, we had no idea about, we will find behind there our own divine potential, that had to be forgotten and renounced. This is precisely, why it is so important to identify our own fears. They reveal the direct path to our own misconceptions, as well as to those shared by society and collectives. Moreover, they reveal the path to our collective true potential and self.

3. From the Fear of Poverty to Wealth

Poverty is the opposite of wealth or prosperity. Interestingly, the German word for poverty is "Armut", which means "lack" or "deficiency". But literally spoken „Arm" in German is „poor" and „Mut" is „courage" - so the literally meaning is „poor of courage". Poverty seems to be at home, where people have not enough courage to re-think their system they are living in. Wealth and poverty stem from the same flow of life and are subject to the same regularities and principles. Until now, however, we have lived under the misconception that poverty equals failure and wealth or prosperity equals success. Traditionally, poverty has been associated primarily with the loss of material prosperity, which is the logical consequence of our current definition of success. However, poverty is much more than that, and the opportunities hidden within it become clear, when viewed from a new perspective of success.

The Fear of Poverty

The fear of poverty exists wherever we are lacking the courage to allow new thoughts, in other words wherever attitudes and values are not questioned. It exists wherever old valuations and the corresponding assessments and judgments, as well as prejudices, cannot be let go of. The word judgment is used here in the sense of appraisal and disdain of a person or thing, based on a lack of awareness. Contrary to pure assessment, judgment is not neutral, but contains disdain and denigration. In German pure assessment is named as „Ur-Teil", which means: „the original or true thing" in its literally sense. Real Judgments are based on fear and lack, whereby the fear always disguises one thing: our "true thing", or the truth of our origin, that lives in everything. This "true thing" is the innermost core, the primal energy; it is love and life. When we fail to recognize this core essence because of the fear of poverty, whether in other people, situations, things, or in ourselves, lack arises with all of its consequences, such as we are witness to today. This fear is like a chameleon: it is so adept at disguising itself, becoming an invisible part of the inner jungle, that it can be carried as a burden throughout an entire life – or even an entire human history – without ever being recognized. The growing number of people that have the courage for honest self-reflection are however allowing us to become aware of this heavy baggage that we have believed to be a part of us.

Poverty

The fear of poverty stems from the fear of being hurt, of being less or less liked, of being small or being made small. We have often experienced life in this. When one suffers from the fear of poverty, they are not generally willing to give or share without condition – regardless of whether material or immaterial. A lack of faith in life itself, along with the learned skeptical belief, that we rarely get anything good in return, when we give of our child-selves out of pure pleasure and the joy of life, are responsible for this fear. We attempt to hoard, collect or multiply, without ever achieving true happiness. And when something akin to success does arise, it is often unknowingly at the expense of others. Particularly in what we call first-world countries, the fear of poverty prompts people to jump onto the proverbial hamster wheel of insatiability. We have a permanent drive to consistently do more and have more, rarely or never finding satisfaction and peace of mind.

Interestingly, we sometimes discover something fascinating when we encounter people that are materially poor. They are often much happier with the little that they have, and even gladly share their humble possessions. Ironically enough, we try to convince these "less fortunate" people, that live predominately in the so-called third world, that they would be happier with our way of life. All the while we are living proof that this concept is dubious or at the very least should be questioned. Could it be, that in reality it is exactly the other way around, and that we could possibly learn something from them, and that everyone concerned would be happier if we could sensibly combine the two approaches?

Anyone who has ever willingly chosen to break loose from the prosperity cycle and renounce worldly pleasures knows, how liberating this is. This example teaches us something: it is important to know what type of prosperity we are striving for, in what way we wish to experience prosperity and how much of it we wish to experience it. These factors are directly correlated to our own motivation. If the fear of poverty is our motivation, or our "why" – whether we are aware of it or not – we will sooner or later experience about as much success as an ant trying to move a boulder. It will be virtually unavoidable that we experience poverty. Whether it is material or psychological/emotional makes no difference – we will experience poverty. This can manifest in many different ways: the loss of material goods, a war of roses over some material issue, or perhaps an illness that results in the inability to work. On a global level we might experience an economic meltdown, an environmental catastrophe, or a cataclysmic war. If, on the other hand, our motivation is the expression of the knowledge of our true nature as divine creatures of love, we will receive the opportunity to transform the above-mentioned challenges – with us and through us.

The Fear of Poverty Rules the World

The fear of poverty manifests itself not only in the lives of each one of us – as a society, we are also increasingly experiencing the consequences of this fear that has been completely hidden from our view, for it seems to reach far beyond our customary interpretation of consciousness and success.

Calculation – in the literal sense of the word – seems to be the core of the problem here, which is inherent in our entire societal system. Debit and credit stand ubiquitously in opposition to one another, like two titans in an eternal battle. When the credit is strong and growing, we experience positive attention and recognition, and we receive more opportunities. When the credit is weak, or if it consists solely of debits, things typically look exactly the opposite. The market for books, lectures and seminars that promise to teach anyone how to attain great riches, is growing at a rapid pace. Some of them advocate and teach the use of methods such as legal loopholes, cheap labor in the Far East, as well as other questionable practices. These things work, of course, on the basis of our current economic and financial systems, and on the basis of what we define as success. They do not, however, create a win-win situation. Not all parties benefit from these practices. More importantly, someone always loses here. This system primarily targets profit; in other words, quantity, but rarely quality. Other people suffer, as well as the environment.

If we dare to take a critical look behind our economic systems, we can discover, how the fear of poverty works. As a relict of our childhood, it prompts us again and again to betray our connection to ourselves, so that we may retain the way in which we have learned to define as positive success. It is this fear that keeps our world economy afloat, although we sense, that something is just not right. Here is one example:

We produce backlogs of goods, although today all goods of this world could be made available to everyone within a very short time thanks to our technological achievements. Meanwhile we are capable of transporting food nearly fresh from one end of the earth to the other. Nonetheless, backlogs of products are produced, only to have their shelf life increased or to be canned. Manipulative technologies are developed to increase the shelf life of our foods or to protect them from the pests that have spread or even evolved through over-cultivation, monocultures and pesticides. All of this and more happens out of fear that an event might someday take place that would necessitate this kind of stockpiling. Here again we can recognize a relict from our ancestors' experience of the world wars.

It is unbelievable yet true: we are destroying biological diversity and our basic food resources, and secondarily even our climate, out of fear that we someday might have nothing left to eat. To feel positive with this way of acting, we defined this as something, that shows the graduation of prosperity, unconsciously covering the fear of loss. But somehow we remain blind to the fact, that we ourselves are destroying our resources. We are provoking the dreaded scenarios of deficiency ourselves through our mindless behavior. In the course of such a cycle, shortage scenarios appear that could easily lead to conflicts on a political level. At that point, food and biodiversity are no longer the focus of the deficiency; it is replaced by the question as to how riches – and with them power – can be secured through commodities, with the intention of winning. We can see that the same cycles repeat again and again, and far too often the welfare of people, animals and the environment is sacrificed for the sake of power and success. And although we are actually adding changes to our agenda with increasing regularity, profit remains so fixed in our sights, that the implemented solutions resemble a drop in the ocean, or the attempt to solve a problem ends up creating numerous new problems.

It is the principle of competition that governs our world, and this principle is rooted in the fear of poverty. If we take the entire gamut of factors into consideration, however, we see that in the end there can be only losers and not a single winner, if we do not reflect upon and express all, that humanity could be in its entirety. We face disastrous consequences, if we fail to do this. On the other hand, the opportunities are grandiose, if we choose to recollect and "primember".

As long as humanity as a whole believes, that competition will move us forward, and we continue working at increasing our wealth through production and invention, and this is not based on self-love, true consciousness, awareness and love for everything that is, it cannot be a blessing for us; it can only be a curse.

Different Thoughts Create Different Circumstances

Let us instead imagine, just for a moment, a radically opposite scenario. We understand that there is no necessity for mass cultivation or genetic manipulation of food, and that nature provides us with everything we need. It is possible today to feed everyone in a short time. What we already have, could eliminate hunger in the world within a short period of time, and far less of our time than would be necessary, to continue generating the masses of food we are currently producing. More time would be left over for physical and psychological wellbeing, which would in turn lead to an easier and faster consciousness. All people would then be able to come together, each in an improved physical and mental state, to reflect upon, how each of us could contribute their calling and transform this earth to the one, most of us obviously want: a peaceful and intact place. Self-love is always accompanied by self-commitment, self-responsibility, self-confidence and one's own purpose.

Anyone that has ventured down the path to self-awareness will know, what he or she can contribute toward making this peaceful, healthy planet a reality. Peace and health begin in each individual – regardless of whether they are from the first world or the third world.
If we want to solve the challenges of our time in a truly meaningful manner, we would be well advised to let go of competition and struggle. Cooperation and kindness are the signposts of our time. The following quote from Prof. Dr. Dan Siegel points directly to the fact, we have apparently forgotten: *"Our present state of scientific knowledge suggests that we can solidly affirm that kindness and compassion are to the brain*

what the breath is to life." Kindness and compassion are based on understanding. The type of understanding referred to here, however, lay far beyond to what is normally available to us within our usual frame of reference. We will receive more insights of our human compassion and full understanding in the course of this book, particularly in the chapters "Understanding" and "Self-Awareness".

New Ways of Thinking – True Values

The erroneous definition of success appears to have led to a scenario where we are mentally chained to prosperity and until now have subconsciously identified ourselves almost exclusively on the basis of our prosperity. But what would remain of us prosperous people, if we were to suddenly lose our riches? What inner riches in terms of security and trust would be present? What would happen, if everything should lose its value? The next question that arises is: why, then, do we hold on so tightly to our old value systems?

National debt is piling up like dry leaves in autumn. What keeps us from adopting new values in place of the old? Why do we not draw a line of demarcation, set all debts – public and private, in an inner and an outer frame – to zero and start anew? What holds us back from developing kindness and compassion beyond the borders of our definition of success? Why do we not finally define new measures of value? Ultimately, at some point in the past somebody simply determined what success, prosperity and wealth mean, what we should consider valuable, and that there must be something like wrongdoing and retribution. The mass of people simply inherited these values, who some people has defined.
If we truly want equality, I can only hope for us all that we (pri-)remember ourselves and undertake such a change intentionally and as an expression of our true selves. Otherwise the laws of the universe and our subconscious will make sure that

our actions sooner or later lead to an automatic reset anyway. The crash scenarios could become reality, although this is not at all necessary. On the other hand, such a crash can also be quite useful: a crash could allow us to introduce a new currency: life time.

Actually, this currency is not so new. Technically speaking, it is already in use – unfortunately, however, more as a curse than as a blessing. Currently people give their life time away for an extremely low value per hour. Here again we can recognize our "quantity over quality" example from earlier. What would it be like if every hour of life time had the same exact value?

Every person on this entire planet has exactly the same 24 hours of life time each day.

If we truly want to speak of EQUALity, we probably won't be able to avoid confronting the consequences that are still very uncomfortable for us – those consequences that do not harmonize with our current definition of success. What does equality mean? Each person is on par with everyone else; no one is better or worse than another. Prosperity would not be possible without the "base and servile" work currently held in such low esteem – we would plunge into chaos.

Our current knowledge and change processes would remain invisible, if we all would not play precisely the role that we are currently playing. It is both visible - what works, as well as what does not serve us. Therefore, everyone and everything would be equally right and important.

A different interpretation of success based on win-win and our divine universal origin would enable us to find solutions and measures that we simply cannot see or allow at present.

Money as a Mirror

Instead of a neutral means of exchange, our relationship to money is an allegory of how we learned to love. Our relationship to money reflects, how our inner horse-trading with and against ourselves and our shares, is handled. If we redefine love and its value by letting go of old misconceptions that have led to fears and vulnerabilities, we can find keys hidden in this change of conviction and behavior, that can be applied to transform our financial and economic systems, and with that, the world. All mechanisms that are found and applied in every individual, are anchored and active in our environment and in the entire world, because all life is subject to the same principles and laws - because all is one.

Our relationship to money is an allegory of our outdated approach to love, coupled as it is with conditions. When you give, you get something in return. When that something does not meet the expectations, then we get less or nothing in return, and if we don't agree, then... Often, two parties understand each other perfectly in the beginning. Then suddenly one party wants more or something different. In a marriage, "not feeling seen, loved or noticed" is far too often carried out as a "war of the roses" at the expense of the children. People argue about material things, whereas what is really missing – the flow of love or understanding– is no longer available. Money seems to be, so to speak, the force behind the love.

We can observe a comparable dynamic in companies, where a similar scenario often develops out of what began as a good partnership due to an accumulation of misunderstandings. If we look on a global level, the greed for commodities or natural resources and the associated greed for power seem to have priority. It was the same procedure centuries ago. Humankind subconsciously operates on the following principle: make an enemy of those from whom you want something, so that you can declare war against them. If at first it doesn't work, we tweak the details of the enemy image until the person or people in question fit the image. This principle impacts us on a personal, societal and global level. It is the fear of poverty that has led us running on this hamster wheel of external and internal compulsions, destroys childhoods through revoking relationships, ruins marriages, causes business failures, promotes arguments between partners – personal and business, and on a grand scale leads to wars and to the destruction of nature and the planet.

What would happen if people simply stopp playing along? Imagine, if there were enough people that are aware of their own responsibility, see through these power and money political games and no longer allow themselves to be led astray by them, in keeping with the motto, "Someday they'll have a war and nobody will come!" Instead we challenge the parties involved to work with true peace mediators to resolve the cause of the misunderstandings, or even to resolve their personal differences man to man. Would they then still want to make war? The same principle could be applied to all existing financial, economic and political systems.

What changes would be possible, if we had the courage to say "no" to all of the things we are feeling the "no" for a long time? The failure to do this until now has allowed the world to come to what we are seeing now. How would it look like in future, if we removed ourselves from these machinations that could not function without us, and defined a new conceptual framework?

Finding the Answers

All that is necessary for a fundamental transformation can be found within each of us. When we disband the fears discussed here and regain the ability to tap the potential hidden behind it, healing on all levels follows – healing for us human beings and healing for the entire planet, for we treat others and our environment in exactly the same manner, that we treat ourselves. We influence each other. When we are at peace with ourselves, we pass this on to others with every interaction. The answers are all there, waiting for us to declare that, if we are ready to recognize ourselves. At that point we are able to recognize, understand and adopt the signposts and guidance that reside inside us, in our environment and in nature, the way they are actually meant. We will no longer manipulate and exploit ourselves or our environment.

This in no way means, that all financial and economic systems must necessarily be abolished, rather, that we simply need new value systems and new perspectives regarding the procedures of our systems. Together we can avert the currently predictable scenarios, if we as humanity are ready to actively bring about changes. If we continue doing what we are currently doing, however, life itself will present us with the next catastrophe as a response to our actions, forcing us to make some change.

The fear of poverty appears on all levels of human being: intellectual poverty, financial poverty, lack of esteem, lack of love, lack of approval, lack of inspiration, lack of joy, etc. It is our greatest burden and simultaneously our greatest gift. If every individual can change their valuations and transform the valuation of fear into the valuation of love, the fear of poverty becomes obsolete.

We, as a collective, have the opportunity to actively bring about the transformation we desire, if each of us begins with ourselves – continuously, step by step, again and again becoming the next better version of our self. Self-responsible thinking and acting grow on the soil of healed wounds and recognized misconceptions. Love always has the best possible outcome for all involved in mind. That is our true nature.

We don't need to fight all these crises, or to discover how to emerge from them in the most advantageous manner. What we need are new values. Until now we have missed the mark with our interpretations and our evaluations. I use the word "missed" intentionally here: we are missing a crucial fundamental factor, namely the responsibility to create a win-win out of every situation. This is the foundation of the heart and the divine core within each of us.

Each of us carries within himself an economic-ethical basis of valuation. We often sense this basis; however, we have also misinterpreted this gift. The more we turn inward and uncover our fears, the more we automatically become aware of this basis and its meaning. The need to consciously experience, what we have hitherto only sensed, arises. If we fail to do this, we experience emotional pain – here lays the subconscious root of our rapidly increasing cases of depression, burnouts and violent acts. We don't understand, where the pain comes from and what its actual purpose is. The responsibility we all share is greater than we ever realized, yet so are our possibilities and potential.

We are the crown of creation for good reason. It was also for good reason that Christ once said, *"The greatest among you will be your servant."* When we look at the role allocation here on earth, however, there is not much to be seen in the way of service. The preservation of our planet is our responsibility. We carry this responsibility with joy, when we recognize the answer within us – the answer to the question of who we truly are. At this point then, we are firmly grounded in our divine universal origin, and we have built solidly, like a rock that can withstand anything, rather than on the sand of misguided success and riches, that is destined to collapse sooner or later. Then we experience true prosperity and wealth on all levels.

4. From the Fear of Illness to Health

The fear of illness has various ramifications and is basically the fear of the loss of health. The primary goal of our actions then should be to maintain or restore health in human beings and our entire environment. This would make sense. As we can see plainly, we take this into account maximum superficially.

Lifestyle Diseases of Today

Lifestyle diseases can be divided into two categories: physical and psychological. The direct effects of physical disease can include lack of productivity, pain, and a wide variety of physical limitations. Known indirect effects include financial and social dependency, and the loss of freedom. As a consequence, self-esteem is impacted.

An increasing number of people are suffering from obesity, cardio-vascular diseases and their effects, diabetes and cancer. The continuous escalation of these diseases alone gives rise to thought. When we consider, however, the increasing occurrence of psychological problems such as depression and burnout, it appears as though it may be time to confront the problem on a different level than simply the physical-psychological. I will intentionally refrain from discussing physical diseases, since the way through the psychological diseases can also result in solutions to the physical diseases that we currently would not deem possible. In any case, we can come to the conclusion that if children and young adults are already suffering from obesity, diabetes, ADHS, depression or burnout, something is direly amiss. Apparently we in the first world are living a lifestyle that is neither beneficial for our bodies nor our minds. When we examine the lifestyle of today, we can easily see that we have created a multitude of factors that promote illness or are an obstacle to the maintenance or restoration of our health. These factors are far removed from our healthcare system.

We live in a state of relatively extreme financial prosperity. We are often fully unaware of this fact, because our standards have risen so rapidly and continue to rise, that we still experience lack in spite of this abundance. The drive for change, improvement and simplification leads to ever more rapid progress, which on the one hand we search for and long to share, and on the other hand seems to be the root of our diseases.

Causes

In the following considerations I am intentionally exploring a larger context beyond the background of conventional medicine, since it is in the framework of that larger context, that new perspectives and with them new solution approaches can be found.

Let us examine the growing variety of food products in our supermarkets. The quantity, e.g. the amount of variety, is continuously expanding, while the quality seems to slip further and further into the background. Often a modern food product does not deserve to be called food. Products are manufactured and advertised, that are obviously not healthy yet continue to find more and more room on the shelves of our stores.

We all know, that sugar in its various forms is not especially beneficial, particularly for children, but also for adults. Nonetheless, a seemingly endless stream of new varieties of sweets is produced and new sweet beverages introduced, which are of course more likely to be chosen than healthy food and beverages. No wonder, then, that more and more children are suffering from obesity and other accompanying symptoms of massive sugar consumption.

The daily rat race prompts an increasing number of people to fall back on ready-made meals, since enough time seems to be absence – and for many people, money does not allow healthy shopping or healthy cooking. Add to this, the dwindling amount of physical exercise, which is supported by this trend. As a cofactor, a lack of exercise also promotes depression, since movement causes the body to release endogenous happiness hormones that are lacking in depression. People rather hide behind our digital media than face all the "crap" out there in the world again. There is also the growing possibility of manufacturing drugs, for example alcohol, in a way that it tastes good and is easy to acquire. After all, drugs of any kind make it easier to cope with all the "crap" out there.

In our adult world, we add the pressure to perform and work conditions to the lack of movement, lack of time and emotional challenges – all that leads to physical and psychological disease. It seems unnecessary to delve into further aspects here, since they all lead us to the same questions: Why are we and our elected governments continuously discussing the fact that our health is barely (or no longer) fundable, while allowing economic developments that create obstacles to our goal of health? How can it be, that products are manufactured that are clearly hazardous to health, and in spite of that, still find their way into our stores – with prices that are lower than the foods that actually deserve to be called foods? How can it be, that a variety of ingredients are not required to be listed simply because they are present in amounts, that are below the legal limit, and that this limit can be adjusted, so that those ingredients never exceed it? How can it be, that we have conditions that allow the level of emotional pressure in schools and the workplace to continually rise? How can it be, that over and over again, conditions are ALLOWED to emerge, that stand in opposition to our goal of health? It seems as though the fear of poverty prevails over the fear of illness, and that we would rather accept illness than to refrain from that, which we believe will lead to success.

Apparently the fear of illness plays a rather insignificant role for many people. This may be due to the fact that illness is often something that emerges slowly and insidiously, and which we hope will strike others, while material failure usually has a quick or immediate impact. The fear of illness, or loss of health, is then abruptly in any person's awareness – whether poor or wealthy – when an actual or impending loss of health threatens that person's productivity and consequently their income.

Expanding our Perception

One extremely interesting aspect of the fear of a loss of health is not the actual loss itself, but the often long-lasting presence of uncomfortable sensations in the absence of any justifiable, visible or understandable physical causes. Several years ago people suffering from this phenomenon were considered hypochondriacs, a condition based on fear. According to Wikipedia, *hypochondria is the worry about having a serious illness; ...the result of an inaccurate perception of the condition of the body or the mind despite the absence of an actual medical condition...* But hypochondriasis is also a symptom, that occurs in numerous psychiatric disorders. These disorders include depression and burnout, which are on the rise.

Let us focus more closely on precisely these disorders for a bit. Basically, one can say that, as long as nothing can be diagnosed physically, a shift in the mindset can reduce the sensations and fears increasingly over time, and health can be quickly restored from the inside, out by rethinking and changing one's own expression of life. People that suffer from such fears are often accused of having an overactive imagination about the worst possible scenario. This is absolutely true. These disorders tend to prevent us from living the life we led previously, and for good reason (albeit previously never appreciated) – they want to show us that the life we led previously no longer serves us.

Sensitivity

What has been overlooked until now is an extreme sensitivity for the "ill", misinterpreted internal realm. One could say, that while these uncomfortable sensations and sometimes overwhelming internal fears are powerfully experienced, their meaning is generally misunderstood. The affected person is neither paid attention to nor taken seriously, since these fears are seemingly irrational and cannot be explained inside of our existing worldview. Everyday life maneuvers the person more and more into the fear, which must be subdued with medications. Often the body must eventually become truly ill, unless a significant change in the habits, that caused this misery, takes place. Its cry for help cannot be answered due to a lack of awareness. We can be grateful, that the body acts as a perfect measuring instrument, indicating any "illnesses" of the mind, that manifests as an expression of a spiritual imbalance. The opportunity lay in the absence of a physical cause. A solution approach can be found in the internal realm, where the cause originated.

What is important here is to take heed of the fact, that the number of people who are struggling with depression and burnout – more and more often at a young age – is increasing rapidly. According to the extensive research of several sources undertaken during the writing of bestselling author Arianna Huffington's book, Thrive: The Third Metric to Redefining Success and Creating a Life of Well-Being, Wisdom and Wonder, the quantity of prescribed anti-depressants in Germany grew 46% between 2007 and 2011; in the USA an increase of 400% since 2008 has been recorded. Over-the-counter, natural and anti-depressive drugs are not included in these statistics. The number of sick days attributed to psychological disorders in Germany rose 80% between 1996 and 2011.
What is this trying to tell us? It seems entirely possible that this development wants to show us, that it is not our fears that are "wrong", but the increasingly unhealthy lifestyles, that we are

currently leading. The fears and the associated illnesses are trying to wake us up, before we become seriously physically ill. Unfortunately, we are living in a world, where many, many people profit financially and materially from illness, and in which apparently not enough money is available to maintain or restore health. Preventative healthcare is still a lower priority than the treatment of illnesses – a fact that we are reminded of daily through the policies of our health insurance carriers. Political and economic policies that represent obstacles to health continue to be supported or not opposed. Given these actualities, the question as to whether we truly wish to be and live healthy is certainly justified. Is this truly our endeavor, or are our efforts really just a way to ease our guilty conscience, so that we can continue to put profit ahead of health. We are living in a time in which we should finally begin to ask ourselves which spirits we are calling and which we have called in the past.

For reasons that will soon become clear, I would like to remind us of the story I quoted earlier about the battle with the flu epidemic in New York during the First World War. The success lay in the fact that the citizens' fear was no longer nourished. The healing followed automatically, because the focus shifted from their fear to mastering their everyday routine with all of its challenges. The people were then solution-oriented rather than fixated on problems. Now, we could say, "So let's just forget the fear and depression and focus on our everyday life." Sure, but the question is, what are the actual and real challenges that need to be mastered? Our daily routine, in its current form, does not seem to deliver these challenges, unless we assume that the routine itself must be changed in a whole new way. When we look around us, we could come to the conclusion that there is plenty to be mastered in addition to the lifestyle diseases – both physical and psychological – that are running rampant, and that we ourselves create in their entirety.
It appears that a new and important factor comes into play here, which was coined by world-renowned author, Neale

Donald Walsh. This approach can facilitate a significantly larger perspective, and is expressed thus: *"It's not about you."* What does this mean? If we turn our focus from our own problems to the examination of all these conditions which led us to these continuously growing wave of disease, it finally becomes clear, that something is amiss in the great overall context, and that we have created a great number of things, that do not serve us or that make us ill. It could become clear that our lifestyle not only endangers the overall balance of each individual, but of the entire planet, and everything that exists on it, and that the whole thing is a cycle of reciprocal inducement.

In Zen Buddhism litterature we find the following tale:
"A wise old man once sat under a tree as the god of plague came along the path. The wise man asked him, "Where are you going?" The god of plague answered, "I am going to the city and will kill 100 people." On his return route, the god of plague once again came along the wise man's path. The wise man said, "You told me you were going to kill 100 people. Travelers reported to me that 10,000 people died." The god of plague responded, "I killed only 100. The others were killed by their own fear."

Our greatest plague is our belief in what we call success. Our subconscious fear of material loss runs so deep, that we are not aware of the rat race we have created because of it; a rat race that – metaphorically speaking – turns the 100 deaths from the tale above into 10,000. The number of people that fall victim to this vicious circle rises daily.

Characteristics of This Fear

The repetition of illness-related complaints is an unnoticed companion in our daily routine. Examples include, "I'm so stressed out", "I don't feel well", "I'm tired", "I'm in so much pain", "I might go nuts if…", "It's driving me insane", and many more. This is accompanied by a total lack of awareness that these complaints draw fear and its consequences more and more into our reality. The continuous repetition of these thoughts or words exacerbates the negative effect. We discuss the issue at length, come up with and invent and try everything imaginable that might bring healing, all with no real success, because scarcely anything is done about the true source of the problem. Subconsciously, the attention that the ailment causes is worth more than an actual change and recovery. Plus, we still profit too heavily financially and economically to want to change anything, since we are not really aware of these interactions. This attention is necessary for us to recognize, that our current attempts at change and recovery are not in alignment with our divine universal truth.

If we look more closely we can surmise a search here. There appears to be a great longing – a longing for… for what? There seems to be in each of us a deep fear carried within and despair that perhaps neither we nor our environment is aware of. In the end, this despair drives us to create solutions for our challenges the same way that we have created them until now. For the sake of perception expansion, here is included an excerpt on the side benefits of. First we will discuss the core issue on the basis of the text, then examine what the consequences look like for the individual and, figuratively speaking, for society.

Despair reduces the sense of guilt, because it feels like a form of penance.
Despair brings sympathy from others—and this sympathy can often feel like love.
Despair justifies abandoning relationships with family and friends with the idea, that they will be better off without the desperate person. Despair is an excuse for avoiding obligations and responsibilities.
Despair is a way of punishing others who feel, they must help and yet fail to help.
Despair makes it difficult for significant others to leave, because

it would mean abandoning a desperate person.
Despair justifies indulging in addictions and other self-destructive but pleasurable behaviors.
Despair, especially when it comes together with the threat of suicide, is a way to dominate others who, afraid to upset the desperate person, will walk on eggshells.

Catch-22 of Despair

While despair gives a sense of doing penance, it is also a way to justify avoiding responsibility. While it brings sympathy, it is also a way of punishing others. While it justifies abandoning relationships, it also makes it difficult for people to leave the person in despair. In this list the inner conflict between the longing for connection and the apparent inability to experience connection the way one wishes to reveals itself. At the core are the connection and the HOW of the connection. By implication, the fear behind it, being incapable of experiencing connection and thus life the way we feel and we want to experience it, also becomes visible. In a wider context, connection not only refers to the connection between us human beings, but also the way that we treat ourselves, others, health and the whole environment and planet. As we have established, the appropriate way of being has been trained out of us, leading to disavowal and separation from the connection to ourselves. As a result, we experience "negative success" in those areas where we feel disconnected with ourselves, reflected in our entire environment. It is the fear of being alone, the separation, that we are repeatedly experiencing anew. The life that most of us are accustomed to living prohibits us from experiencing being one in love with everything – the experience of our true selves, which presupposes this connection to one's self.

A lack of "inner exercise" as a sign of inner rigidity and inflexibility of our thoughts and beliefs, is the result of this phenomenon. As a consequence, our physical and – more importantly – inner, "mental-spiritual" immune system, or the ethics of our soul, shuts down. This process is further supported by negative thoughts and words. The body's energy level declines incessantly, and the susceptibility to illnesses of all kinds increases. Financial worries and lack of time are common side effects. Important tasks are not completed, or never started, and cannot be completed later if illness follows – a disastrous cycle that feeds itself. Excessive use of pain medications, alcohol and other medications, drugs, as well as work and digital media, serve to superficially subdue or dull the symptoms.

At this point we now interpret the aspects of individual despair as described in a wider context. When we examine the individual aspects of despair, it becomes clear, that this instrument is also utilized on a political level. The desperate attempts to attain new acquisitions and methods for changing that, which we originally brought about ourselves, reduces the sense of guilt. The election campaigns are rife with exaggerated promises that cannot be agreed upon by the majority after election. The extent to which we live for success separates us evermore from the connection to ourselves, our partners, our children, and our families. This devastating hamster wheel keeps us from meeting necessary obligations for long-overdue consequences. A change could mean letting go of all of the prosperity and imagined security, that we have grown so attached to, so it seems more sensible to regulate more and punish those, who allegedly oppose our success structure, than to implement true change.

More and more addictions and addictive substances are being created and in some ways even subconsciously promoted, and the self-destruction of man and nature advanced; since no escape is visible, this seems like the easiest way. The threat of an impending financial and economic collapse as a symbol of suicide, with all its hideous consequences and the subsequent suffering, still works its magic, keeping us strapped to the hamster wheel and pedaling furiously. The minor rectification agreements and renaturation measures occur to us as penitence, yet in the context of the greater responsibility they are nothing more than the proverbial drop in the ocean.

The aforementioned lack of "inner exercise" as a sign of inner rigidity and inflexibility of our thoughts and beliefs becomes visible through the endless political and economic debates, that take place without any of the improvements that are necessary for humanity and the environment. The immune system of the society is shut down, supported by the negative thoughts and words of the people themselves. People are so preoccupied with mastering the challenges of the hamster wheel, that the event that would serve as an immune system, can no longer come to pass. The energy level of the society sinks incessantly. The susceptibility to "failure" (rise in illness, corporate bankruptcies, violent demonstrations, etc.) rises. Financial worries and lack of time are common side effects. Important tasks are not completed, or never started, and cannot be completed later if "failures" (natural catastrophes, financial or economic crash, war, epidemics, terror, etc.) follow – a disastrous cycle that feeds itself. Excessive use of all sorts of wonderful luxury goods and habits serve to superficially subdue or dull the symptoms.

The Pursuit of Happiness

Inner distress, as well as curiosity and imagination, of the increasing number of people falling ill, lead to an excessive amount of research on the Internet and study of the correlated challenges. The pursuit of happiness in life is in the foreground. It seems to be that we will end up owing a great deal to these people who suffer extremely under the fear of the loss of health. Every single one of them has contributed to an infinite wealth of knowledge and experience, and cleared the path to new avenues, through their propensity toward research and testing of numerous healing methods. These people uncover all the ways that we are subconsciously harming ourselves. Whether it is our consumption of foods that are not good for us, or behaviors that are required of us in spite of their detrimental consequences, because societal norms stipulate them. The old ways no longer work, yet measured by our current standards, the new ways do not appear to offer any acceptable alternatives that lead to a truly healthy lifestyle. It looks as though it is time to question our current standards and at the very least consider the possibility, that we urgently need new standard and new measures of value.

Perception of Health and Illness

There have been several interesting experiments on the topic of our psychological-energetic immune system. It was discovered that, in the majority of cases, if a perfectly healthy person is continuously told by the people around them how terrible or sick they look, they will fall ill within a short amount of time. The fear of illness has set its foot in the door; the person in question let it in. This phenomenon is based on the following mechanism: The perceptions brought in from the outside are adopted and accepted as true. Repetition exacerbates the effect. At this point it is no longer necessary for anyone to forward the action from the outside. We take on the task ourselves of our own free will, believing what the outside people told us. We have learned to trust the perceptions from outside more than those from inside of us.
This contains two interesting and eminently crucial messages: We have learned to trust our perception of the bad or disadvantageous, as well as things that are not aligned with our true self, more than we trust ourselves. We mistrust most positive things that come from the outside. "That's too good to be true" or "Where's the catch?" are statements that express this mistrust – a remnant of our past experiences.

The Key

Now we want to examine the two above-mentioned points very closely, and reverse the valuation standard of the respective context. For each of us individually this means to closely scrutinize what is actually positive and what is not, seen from a new definition of success that is aligned with our true origin. It is possible that we end up believing the great promises of today's success society in regard to material wealth and the pursuit of happiness less, than the results of the scientific research regarding true health and the health of our planet. Things that serve temporary satisfaction can no longer be chosen in place of the long-term retention of health, since this will sooner or later lead to an increasingly disastrous cycle.

A shift in perception can show us what is truly negative in the sense of not serving life or us, and what is truly positive in the sense of serving life and us. The key is to allow that, which will create balance between the promises and the scientific research results mentioned above in a way that benefits everyone and everything. The answer lay within us. The inner resistance that leads to illness is a sign from our soul that our life does not represent the real truth about life. The body, as a means of expression for the soul, is rebelling.

When we place our own universal purpose ahead of our familiar success-oriented thinking, we can apply this mechanism in a truly meaningful and beneficial manner. This mechanism is not bad – it is only wrong in the sense of being applied in a way, that don't serve us. It is time for us to use this very same mechanism FOR OURSELVES and not only for profit.

Crisis or Opportunity?

"A crisis is a productive state. You simply have to get rid of its aftertaste of catastrophe." This quote from Max Frisch points

directly to our dualistic interpretation of a crisis: fear sees a crisis as a catastrophe, while love sees an opportunity for change. This does not mean, that a positive mindset makes us immune to crises. Love would, however, in this case perceive a crisis with trust and openness as an opportunity for growth, searching the solutions in love. When one sows seeds to a crisis out of worry, fear and faintheartedness will not choose the path of openness ahead, but rather the path of reticence and fear behind. We say „NO" to the things, which are already here and therefore we are not able to find and use the chance of insight and growth, because we overlook the concurrent causes.

This has consequences for human beings specifically and for humanity in general. As long as we are more interested in the generation and temporary enjoyment of profitable activities than in true, long-lasting health of human beings and the environment, we will be hard pressed to establish any real solutions. If we consider, that not only individuals but also the entire world could be ill due to a misconception, we can reasonably assume, that new paths are opening up. Rationally speaking, these new paths would still require economic and financial means; the difference is, that we would be applying them in service of and in alignment with our true selves, rather than against nature and for the destruction of humanity and our environment. The health of each individual is tightly interwoven with the health of humanity, as well as the health of our whole planet. The part of our inner selves that has been ignored for so long is now bringing this to light via fears, disharmony and inner and outer resistance.

Healing Potential

Fully astonishing recoveries are witnessed through the effects of and impetus created by the love of another person – even with people suffering under severe depression. To fall in love with another is to open the door to yourself anew, allowing you to rediscover self-healing powers that were previously hidden from your view. Love truly does dissolve all boundaries, for it reconnects the outer world with the inner self. The human being is reminded of their true self, without being aware of it or of the corresponding opportunities and responsibilities. We will come back to this potential and its meaning in the last chapter.

The love of self brings healing and enables us to realize, that we are connected to everything. If we can eliminate our misconceptions, we can begin to see, that we heal quickly because our true self-awareness would show us, that we were always whole. When we are aware of our true selves, we realize that we always play our part in our own health and the health of the world – whether beneficial or not. The question is whether we will choose our health and the opportunity to experience who we truly are.

5. From the Fear of Death to Living

For many the fear of death is one of the most horrifying fears and it is closely connected to the fear of futility.. Nobody wants to think about death, but behind this fear, there is something extraordinary at play - life! The fear of death is in reality the fear of the loss of life and it has two characteristics: the fear of physical death and the fear of death of the soul.

Physical Death

What is usually at play here, is not the fear of death itself but rather the fear of the manner of dying. We find a connection here to the fear of the loss of health. Most people wish to be healthy until old age in body, mind and soul and then fall asleep or drop dead. Few of us, however, are granted such mercy.
I had several encounters with death during my time as an intensive care nurse, but I will always remember one particular example. A 93-year-old lady was lying in her bed, kept alive by a ventilator. She had suffered a stroke and the odds of her requiring permanent care where extremely high, if not unavoidable altogether. The measures to keep her alive were explained with: "she was walking her dog for a couple of miles every day until the end and she was in great shape – we can't just let her die like that." Several similar and an increasing number of examples like that, followed until now.

A Paradox of Potentials

This part of the book could be a bit challenging for some, and I want to remind you again that this is not about judging but about ascertaining data on a factual level. Day in and day out, people whose lifespan would be over, are prevented from being allowed to die. They are connected to machines without which they could not survive. Old people who do not wish to live any longer, who of their own will stop eating and drinking and are ready to die, are force-fed with tubes and IVs.

Millions upon millions are spent keeping these people alive, yet at the same time we complain about the increasing senescence of society and exploding healthcare costs, that we can no longer afford. We're spending money, which seems to be deficient everywhere.

These people have already given their contribution to life and yet the gift of being allowed to go, is being denied them. At the same time, many thousands of children die each day on our planet from hunger and malnutrition. Roughly 800 children per hour are dying. They are starving to death in a world of abundance. People – children, who never get a chance to give their contribution to this world.

The Analogy

These two examples show, how differently we deal with the topic of death in the rich world and the poor world. We can be grateful, that things are the way they are, because in a metaphorical sense this reflects our acting nowadays. The old and familiar habits and belief systems are being kept alive – at any cost. Habits, convictions and belief patterns are being held on to, although they stopped truly contributing to life, long ago. A great rebellion and a NO resounds from all sides. Insane amounts of money are invested into the "survival" of these habits, convictions and belief patterns, delaying their death, with ever newer and better technologies – yet without any chance of success. On the contrary, this course of action costs us all of our energetic as well as psychological and physical resources. Our reserves are being depleted to the point of overexploitation. In return, we are starving the dreams, potentials and goals of peace and love, we were born and grew up with, to death. If they want to survive, they have to do it on their own. Strangely enough, we expect them to survive without being cared for, nurtured and fed. Is it any wonder then, that more

and more people are suffering, and that our world looks the way it does? We are allowing our own future to starve to death – literally as well as figuratively.
The longer we succumb to our old habits, the more of our life space is taken up by all these fears and their consequences. Life itself becomes increasingly futile.

Visions and dreams have the potential to transform life into the experience it was always meant to be for us. The internal as well as the external Third World contains knowledge and insights, that were missing until now to help restore the balance of the whole. Is it not possible that the challenges of our times could be mastered, if we let go of the belief, that only we in the civilized Western or First World know how everything is supposed to work? A misconception which has, over millennia, led native populations - who knew how to live in harmony with energy and nature - being forced to depart from their ways, if necessary by killing or punishing them, with the result, that we now find ourselves on the brink of total destruction of our planet, unless we stop to reflect and remember our true origin.

The Primordial Lie

Let us now examine the secondary manifestation of this fear. It is the cause of terrorist attacks, wars and executions, as well as genocide, and it is directly related to the previous paragraph. We encounter this manifestation more and more these days. It is the fear of the death of the soul or the fear of the loss of eternal life.
This fear has been nurtured over an eternal period of time up to the present day by a multitude of religions. An eternity is one hell of a long time. So it's not very surprising, that we are determined to secure our ticket to eternal life and heaven at any cost. Religions have gifted us with the misconception, that heaven is waiting for us somewhere and eternal life is waiting

for us sometime. Eternal life is the most powerful leverage, humans can use to exert power and control over others. God is apparently something out there, that is exceedingly mighty and powerful and virtually unrivaled. This separation is, what makes the abuse of power through misinterpretation and thus manipulation possible.

Victims of Religion

These people believe that they have no power, which suffocates criticism nearly immediately, makes reflection much more difficult, and renders personal and individual responsibility virtually impossible. The result is tolerating and not rebelling against the superiors, so as not to jeopardize the salvation of the soul. Instead there is a waiting for a miracle. Most people on earth act like this. This millennia-long religious indoctrination spans like fine cobwebs across the fabric of our societies, although they superficially appear to be losing power and importance. These age-old energies and patterns are embedded in all the structures of our thinking, feeling, speech and actions, and require conscious detection. Those, who allow themselves to cast a glance behind our walls of fear and shadows, will recognize that heaven and the divine, as well as eternal connection and destiny are waiting for us right there. Heaven on earth becomes a reality. It becomes clear that these religious teachings contain valuable messages at their core but have been misinterpreted.

Perpetrators of Religion

Those, who become fighters for religion, disregarding the fact that their fanatic expression has nothing to do with the original message of their religion, do so to their best knowledge and belief and their faith in God. They try to win the salvation of their own soul at any cost. Hiding behind the struggle is, in reality, the fear of loss of eternal life – the worst "punishment" that any soul could ever endure. Add to this, the fear of the futility of our own existence, which drives many to fight so violently for this cause. Characteristic for this group of people is the contempt with which they generally treat women and their expression, granting them few to no rights and using them like objects, that are obligated to be of service. Not only do they abuse women and all people who do not think as they do in the context of their one and only truth, but in doing so, they also demonstrate completely subconsciously, how they misunderstand and abuse their own feminine side and their connection to their divine core and origin. They grew up that way; in their world, this behavior is absolutely normal and proper, since they never experienced anything else. They lack the breadth of perception necessary to see, that this is in no way part of the divine universal order and also inhumane. Now, before one of us slips into judging and condemning, how anyone can possibly think that way, I do wish to simply remind us of the aberrations of Christianity, with its crusades and witch burnings or Christianization of the natives at other continents, which basically represented the same exact dynamic. We Christians, too, were lost, and massively demonstrated exactly the opposite of what has been and is being preached in the Bible as the alleged word of God. It is even said in the Bible: *"for they know not what they do."* It seems quite possible and even logical, that some things were misunderstood or misinterpreted in the transcription of the lore, resulting in a "Chinese whispers" effect. The two following English words provide an excellent metaphorical example of this. The message of Christianity contains the waiting for the return of Jesus Christ, as the son of God, who will take those who are ready with him, so that they shall be where he is, in heaven.

In English "son" means offspring. But there is a word which, when spoken, sounds identical but has a completely different meaning. It is the word "sun", which refers to the celestial body. Could it not be, that at some point in the handing down of the lore, the sun or rather light of God became the son of God?

Could it not be, that we fell prey to a massive misunderstanding in the initial oral tradition, because there may have been words with similar sounds but different meanings? The consequence would be devastating, because our entire view of the world and of success leans consciously or subconsciously on that Christian lore. Suddenly a new meaning emerges when you consider, that the wait for one single and already deceased human, returning sometime in the future brings with itself the fact, that all the divine and universal light in everyone and everything, was the entire time completely overlooked and thus our own being, the presence of the Divine and, with that, heaven on earth could not be recognized. It would suddenly make sense, if we were no longer waiting for the appearance of Jesus Christ, but rather for the appearance, or better, the remembering of the light, that is already there in everyone and everything. It was in fact shining the entire time but we never recognized it as such.

Could this possibly also have exacerbated the effect of the man and the masculine rising above the woman and the feminine as well as everything else in existence, because this interpretation is an automatic and logical but subconscious connection of the masculine figure of God and Jesus the Savior? Could it be, that the one we're waiting for is not a man but simply we altogether ourselves? Human beings, who know all too well the preoccupations and needs as well as the wishes and desires of daily life? Simply human beings, which then are deeply aware of their divine, universal roots and therefore aware of everything surrounding them, wanting to finally clarify all these misunderstandings. For all these confusions and aberrations to this day, we are missing the point, that the goal is not the preservation of power on the outside, but the creation and preservation of self-awareness and self-empowerment on the inside. It is not about God being somewhere or sometime. No – the heart of the matter is the realization that everything humanity has devoured itself for and has fought countless bloody battles and wars for, can be found inside of us. And whoever finds this divine core inside themselves in the form of self-awareness and self-love, and connects and unites with that core, will be allowed to witness all those prophesied miracles here and now on this planet, because they then unite with God or the primal universal force. These persons are no longer able to act contemptuously towards anyone without harming themselves, because it contradicts their ethics of the soul and their knowledge of the divine universal roots in everyone and everything.

Commonality

Common to the "victim" as well as the "perpetrator" is the denial of personal responsibility. The example above about the son and the light or the sun illustrates, why there cannot be any personal responsibility. If one does not know oneself, one cannot give oneself an answer – at least not one that makes any real sense. So the „victim" could lose their sense of personal responsibility for their own visions, dreams and goals, while the „perpetrators" lost their sense of personal responsibility for their acts of violence and atrocities committed in the name of God. Both give up their personal responsibility to God because they succumb to the misconception of the separation from God. The consequence of this is: anything we create out of that context has absolutely nothing to do with the original message of love and divine universal provenance.

Fear of Futility

Perpetrators as well as victims of the fear of the death of the soul seem to regard their role as perpetrator or victim respectively as their purpose in life, which in turn at some point is expected to grant them the opportunity to be reunited with God. How do we move from this misinterpretation to the true meaning of life?

From Futility to the Meaning of Life

The fear of the loss of purpose is something that an increasing number of people in our society are preoccupied with, and which reflects the Zeitgeist of change in this age and time. We can sense, that in everything that surrounds us, including our own existence, there must reside a certain purpose. It seems that material satisfaction is also not the reason we are here, so we must ask ourselves, what then is the meaning of life?
A relatively high level of social justice (in the broadest sense and compared to other countries) and prosperity are present, combined with a similar level of dissatisfaction. This dissatisfaction gives rise to the question of purpose. This dissatisfaction is not the sign of a curse, but rather a blessing for all of humanity. It is the beginning of a longing for change.

Destiny

The fears of the past have lost importance, finally giving space to the fear of the loss of purpose, for that fear shows the path to our destiny. The following examples will illustrate in a simplified manner, what is meant by destiny. It is the destiny of seeds to be put in the earth and bring harvest. It is the destiny of machines to function in a way, that they can be used according to their application. It is the destiny of the individual parts of the machine to work together, to enable the destiny of the machine to be fulfilled. It is the destiny and purpose of our cells and organs to make our physical life possible. WHAT FOR? So that we can fulfill our destiny. The same destiny or purpose, which we have forgotten. What could be our purpose, that we, as the only species on this planet, are equipped with such a refined system of conscious, subconscious and superconscious mind? What is the destiny of all humans on this earth, that we „have to" fulfill together in order to complete something extraordinary bigger than us? Wherein lay the un- or misinterpreted cooperation for the larger purpose of this planet?

The Essential Question

The so called slave driver of our "misconception of success or prosperity" has banished many onto a hamster wheel, thus the question of purpose rightfully enters the space. Many fail at this question, because they either collapse on their hamster wheels or fall into depression, succumb to a burnout or begin to think that they're going crazy. An increasing number of people, including a shockingly increasing number of adolescents and young adults, fail to recognize any reason for their existence or for what surrounds them. They perceive themselves and their environment, and recognize a growing discrepancy between themselves and what exists. The rising number of young people who choose to commit suicide should be an alarm for us. Maybe all these "crazy" kids and young people, who don't seem to subordinate themselves anymore, are not as "crazy" as we think. Maybe they simply unconsciously „know" much better who they truly are and find no conditions, that are a match for their true being. Maybe they have it right, and our system or our demands, evaluations and assessments of what life is supposed to look like, are wrong – not in the moral sense of "wrong" but literally. Like the negative of a photograph does not allow us to properly recognize the motif, and only development through various processes enables us to behold the true image. Something similar seems to be the case, regarding our perception of the world.

We have come to a point where more saber-tooth tigers surround us than ever before: debt crisis, increasing senescence, overpopulation, exploding health care costs, traffic problems, poverty problems, terrorism and war, as well as climate change and environmental disasters. Given all that, it doesn't help much to merely look after our own wellbeing and prosperity. Without a grasp of the big picture, each of us remains as a cog in the clockwork of the entire planet, forever searching. In order to master these challenges, we seem to urgently need one thing: the ORIGINAL mindset, which is rooted in unconditional love. Those who consciously look around themselves realize, how great the longing for peace and love has become. This mindset resides in each human being from the first moment on. Yet it lay buried beneath all the garbage – all the collective and familial thought and belief system junk.

The Journey IS the Destination

Everything that we perceive through our recognitions and experiences along this path reveals to us the reason, why negative things are part of our reality. They all have the right to exist but they needn't to exist any longer. They just want to show us, by way of the feelings we experience through them, what is actually keeping us from our true nature. When we change, they will also change automatically.

Faces of Loss of Purpose

People withdraw more and more and question what is, what was, and what may be. Operating from the old, familiar fear-based worldview, the thoughts that arise will more often than not further nourish the visions of fear. A perpetual feeling of powerlessness takes hold and is accompanied by a sense of futility. If this progresses, we begin to think often about dying, forgetting to make of life, what we came here to make of it. This can go so far, that it becomes a death wish out of a lack of alternatives and goals, even though we only want to live and love. The apt expression cannot be found. This process is accompanied by the feeling of being very much alone, which is virtually unbearable or even devastating. The fear of futility is far more powerful than the fear of the loss of life, because before staying in such a big futility, we CHOOSE death as the best alternative. Being alone – which, out of our erroneous definition and misinterpretation of success leads to separation, lack and loss –

causes us to despair. Herein lays the big jeopardy of our nowadays circle of life. If we step forward like every day in that hamster wheel of success, it is absolutely possible, that humanity will reach one day the point of insight, that it IS better to die and chose distraction, than to continue in this loss futility. And that seems to have happened so many times before, when humanity was in their bloom. They destroyed themselves and their world with all its achievements.

But to be alone out of love is that, which we truly long for: al(l)-one = to be one with all and everything – the feeling we came to the world with. Through despair, life demands of us again and again to take things in our own hands and to remember how everything – and we – really are and were always meant to be.

6. From the Fear of Loneliness to Love

This fear is the greatest fear of all, owing to its depth and origin. On a personal level, it is a breeding ground for jealousy, depression and sometimes paranoia and even suicide. This extremely powerful fear is capable of effectively destroying not only one's own life, but also the lives of others. Herein lays one of ne biggest reasons for the circumstances of our personal as well as global world. Impulsive actions are often at home here. Since the fear of criticism is strongly linked to the fear of being alone, we begin by approaching the topic from that angle.

From „Worrying about" to „take care for" something

Taking care for something is a virtue when properly understood. But this topic also fell prey to a misinterpretation. To take care for something has been confused with worrying about something. To care for something means a providence, as it originates in love, while to worry about something refers to a kind of care that originates from the fear of loss.

Worries and worrying have the characteristic of originating from a lack of trust. The ability of another or of oneself, to take their life into their own hands in an appropriate manner, and to live according to the standards and rules, is subconsciously being disputed. Here the fear of losing a person or thing, that one loves, or the fear this person may come to harm or will be harmed by another person, acting against our rules and standards of our environment, is at play here. Criticism is born.

Criticism

Criticism is the sword, wielded by the fear of loss of love. Unfortunately, we all learned early on to use this sword against ourselves. Not so many years ago, childlike misbehavior was met not only with criticism, but also with beatings. As we can easily imagine, this results in a disdain for criticism. Anyone that was spared corporal consequences is nonetheless familiar with mental and emotional consequences in the form of verbal criticism and withdrawal of love.

Today, we often subconsciously and naturally take over this task, that we learned from our early environment - against ourselves and against others. In spite of all that, criticism was actually born of love, as was revealed in the section "from worrying about to take care for something".

Due to the strong dependence and identification with former persons of reference, we often react to any other person in the same way. It is not clear to us, that it is not love or approval and appreciation that is lost, but rather the connection to oneself, which is erroneously linked to the other person and our false definition of love. It cannot be entirely dismissed that in relationships the withdrawal of love or attention is a means to emphasize our criticism of the other person's way of being. This runs through all relationship structures. Familiar statements such as, "If you don't... then..." bear witness of this. Based on such experiences, it is no surprise, that the fear of the loss of love, thus the fear of aloneness exists, since the natural and individual expression of the relationship with oneself is subconsciously disputed. Criticism becomes a personal affair, that threatens our existence and stands in a way in front of the expression of our true self.

Fear of criticism is the fear from which many branches of the economy thrive. New things or new models of things are constantly designed and sold, which we already own but absolutely "need" to have again in this new and improved form, in order to be happy. If we don't follow these trends, we are certain to experience the criticism of those around us, or even our own internal criticism ("I am worse/less because I can't afford...") in short order. In science and research, we find similar things according to health and the search for or the use of other ways of healing.

The Why and its Consequences

Whether the fashion industry, the automotive industry, electronics industry, health industry or any other industrial branch of design items and even health branches in the broadest sense, they all have one intention: TO SELL.

To this end, new products are continuously introduced to the market. Old and new products trade places every season. Particularly in the area of technology devices, ever-newer products are produced, and no value is placed on repairs any longer. Some electronic devices, are intentionally programmed to display an error message after a predetermined period of time. Similarly, in the fashion industry, new collections are brought out at increasingly short intervals along with the suggestion, that we remain loyal to the hamster wheel of consumption – things are after all getting cheaper and cheaper all the time. Even the health industry works after this pattern, by inventing more and more things to hopefully become healthier without changing any circumstances of life or behaviors. But at whose expense is this all happening? For one thing, at the expense of Mother Earth, who is forced to swallow all of our waste. Secondly, at the expense of less fortunate people – often even children – who do the production work for next to nothing under desolate conditions and unbearably long hours, so that we can always be up-to-date. And thirdly at our own expense, because it is we who continuously keep running on the hamster wheel, searching for prosperity, happiness and security, and who simply keep propelling the existing system faster and more vigorously, even though we are already running out of breath. This does not look like a win-win situation - neither for us ourselves nor for anybody or anything else. We are led to believe that we will be "happier" „healthier" and „more peaceful", if we follow those trends and paths. But the deep-seated desire of humanity to belong, find happiness and to live, has long been abused as strategic sales tool.

Fear of criticism, and more importantly the fear of the consequences of the criticism and the threat of being alone, prompt many people to do things that do not serve them, and have them fall silent instead of doing something about it. Meanwhile, it is the same fear that has us stuck on the hamster wheel of our daily routine in the belief, that following certain guidelines will lead to security, prosperity and growth. We know no other life than the life in this system, yet the consequences of this system beget us an endlessly growing number of physically and mentally ill people, desolate structures of the relationships - couple, families or every other relationship - and conditions on earth, that don't really seem to serve anyone.

The Two Sides of Criticism

The fear of criticism has two sides – the receiving side and the expressing side. Criticism can be very destructive, for it can cause people to stop believing in themselves and their goals, desires, possibilities, abilities and potentials. Fear of criticism can steal all courage to try new things. Our own imagination and creativity is hidden or withers away completely. It curtails individuality, because the goal of criticism is, to make something similar or identical. Independence is dramatically impacted the more often criticism is expressed. The criticized person begins to refrain from doing anything out of the fear of doing the wrong thing. Interestingly enough, we are suffering yet again from an erroneous definition, in this case of the word criticism, with false perceptions and detrimental habits being among the consequences. The word criticism has its origins in the Greek language and came to us by way of the French language. Its original meaning was "to differentiate".

Differentiation

Meaningful and valuable "criticism" is indeed indispensable for growth. Self-criticism, or even external criticism, does not need to be something negative, if we take it as evaluation rather than slipping into judgment. It is time to define criticism newly and to stop demonizing it as something that it actually is not.

Of course, one does not only make friends with criticism of traditional values. Yet precisely herein lay the problem and the solution at the same time. Life is change and it progresses forward continuously. Change is not possible without criticism, since criticism is the evaluation but not the judgement or condemnation of a thing or an action based on defined measures.

The word "measure" appears here as an important factor in our day and age, since a context of fear, power and manipulation is going to apply completely different measures than a context of connectedness, love, health and peace. When we observe the measures that have led to our worldview in the past, we can see that a shift would merely require new measures, which however must be aligned with the universal divine order. Our inherent desire to follow a higher power would be connected with immediate success and most importantly with true purpose, if everyone would simply follow the truly original higher power inside of us all. Suddenly we would have reached the goal not only to make something similar or identical, but we could see everything IS similar and identical, because all is one. It is for good reason that it said in the Bible, *"Let every soul be subject unto the higher powers."* The question does arise, however, as to who the true higher power is and, in the case of a worldly higher power, is it beneath the superiority of „God" or whatever we choose to call the creating energy. Currently I would answer the latter question with an unequivocal NO. The statement from the Bible, *"Fill the earth and subdue it,"* was misunderstood due to a lack of true self-confidence and self-awareness on the part of the secular powers, and thus led to what seems to have already been repeating itself for an eternity. Because one thing went completely forgotten „*The greatest among you shall be your servant of all*". Hatred, war, discontentment and destruction as omnipresent opposites to love and peace bear witness of that misunderstanding.

The Fundamental Flaw

The fear of loss of love often sprouts blossoms, fully unrecognized, in a particular area we are very familiar with: jealousy. The cause for jealousy is a massive lack of trust. It can probably be most easily described on the example of everyday romantic relationships and marriages. Incessant questioning and belaboring the same accusations and suspicions lead to increasingly difficult conditions of daily life together. This false definition of love can have such a disastrous impact, that facts are completely ignored or distorted to fit the reality of the jealous person. There seems to be no desire to find a genuine solution to the core problem. The mistrusted person can say, do or even prove what he or she wants; it will never truly be accepted. Once jealousy has taken hold and burrowed deeper, the jealous person will more and more often become suspicious and find apparent evidence for his or her accusations. Extreme cases of jealousy reach so far, that everything and everyone is under general suspicion, even if there is no reason for it.

The inner fear of the loss of love leads to such immeasurable consequences. The partner under suspicion at some point either sets sail because this suffocating form of love is simply unbearable, or there will rise a fight by hurting each other and try demonstrating the own point of view and power with increasing new methods, or they will give up on themselves in favor of the jealous person. The lack of trust on both sides causes the well of love to dry out. But the jealous person carries much more responsibility for that burdensome situation than they'd like to admit to themselves and more than they are able to realize. This person has, without noticing, played their role in such a perfect way that the worst possible fear is destined to become reality. Eva-Maria Zurhorst describes it very well in her book "Love Yourself and it Doesn't Matter Who You Marry": *"The betrayed person always leaves first."* Since I have been able to gather experience as both, the betraying person and the betrayed person, I can only confirm that statement. Anyone that can truly, openly and honestly reflect upon themselves with all flaws, which are basically just special effects, cannot avoid recognizing and admitting their full responsibility for such a situation, if they want different results.

Digging Deeper

If we look deeply into the core structures of the paragraph above, we can see that similar patterns are at play in commercial, business and political relationships. It seems as if the previous fight for recognition, appreciation and love is now fought unrecognized on all levels of human relationships. Here it is simply no longer jealousy, but rather envy and greed. All sorts of fantastic camouflages, that are deployed with absolutely no conscious awareness, find fertile soil here. The corresponding dynamic to the general suspicion seen in jealousy is, in envy and greed, the excessive controls at airports, that put every traveler under general suspicion of being a terrorist, attempting to bring explosives or weapons onto a plane, just to name an example. For the vast majority of people there is no reason to do such a thing, yet such regulations are created to protect us. The source of these confrontational excesses between terrorists, their organizations and governments can ultimately be found in their struggle for power, which have completely other reasons than these which are shown up. The beginning and real reasons are often completely undiscovered, because we are much too less unaware about the real roots.

Love and money lay closer to each other than we would like, because it is not about them but about relationship. The relationship not only between human beings, but the relationship between everything that exists. If we would really understand our relationship to ourselves, then the logical conclusion would be the understanding of all relations with each and of all that is, because all is one.

A new definition of love, based on the way it truly is, can cure the malaise of misunderstandings at the source. For that which we are currently living is conditional love in all its forms and variations. When we overcome the fear of being alone by allowing constructive criticism of ourselves and our environment, we realize that this false definition of love led to the false definition of success, which in turn caused us to create our world the way it is now. If we can lift that false interpretation we will realize, that we as individuals are and always have been truly one with everything, as we can witness on the condition of this world and everything that lives on it. The fear of being alone can then be replaced by the originally intended experience of being al(l)-one in love.

We will now proceed to the second part of this book, which will shed more light on the most familiar characteristics of success. This will not only show how these things are interconnected and which path can lead us out of our overwhelming disasters, but also make clear that, only together we can win, what we think we lose through change.

Part 2

1. Longing and Desire

Longing and desire is the aggregate that rings in change and turns wishes into their corresponding outer manifestation. The more intense a wish or desire, the more easily it becomes reality. That is why desire is the first step to success; both are the yet somewhat vague beginnings of change.

Status Quo

For a long time, we misunderstood our desire and our yearning for change and the new. This misunderstanding is what led to the conditions we are experiencing today regarding ourselves, our closer and wider environment and the world.
We erroneously sought to fulfill our longing and desire for inner riches outside of ourselves, splitting the world into poor and rich, powerful and helpless. Striving for wealth and more possessions seems to be compensating a lack of love and fullness in heart and the misunderstood connection to our divine nature. This misunderstanding begets further and further misunderstandings, so that we establish desires today, that lead to illness and addiction and destroy our ecological balance within ourselves and on our planet, and we don't seem to know, how to deal with it in a more productive way.
Day to day we feel desires that all too often lead – consciously and subconsciously – to destructive and self-destructive behaviors. Daily „strife and violence" against ourselves and others testify to this.

Effects

I will not go into great detail here, since we already explained this in connection with fear. There is, however, one thing that I wish to repeat.
The desire for external wealth leads to an increasing number of

people being stuck on the hamster wheel, becoming progressively weaker, sicker and unhappier. The additional wealth gained only fills this emptiness superficially if at all. Children are prepared for this rat race in families and schools, and are released into their futures with more and more incidents of behavioral problems, depression, burnout syndrome and a feeling of listlessness or futility.

Other desires appear as a means of compensation. This may be the desire for alcohol, cigarettes, drugs, computer games, social media, television, any kind of luxuries und luxury behavior or whatever may cover up the true, unfulfilled and long unrecognized desire to "be able to be yourself". This substitute desire is sometimes intentionally used to create addictions which will fuel profits. Moreover, this cycle of continuously rising compulsive consumerism and the insatiable desire for more leads to production of our goods in low-wage countries, so that profits continue to increase for a selected few and mass consumption can be guaranteed or even boosted. The conditions allowed by these methods can largely be considered uncivilized – for human beings and for our environment.

Consequences

In our so-called first world, a sense of futility can be found and more and more people are beginning to recognize, that we cannot continue on this way. The deep longing has been visible unconsciously everywhere for quite some time. What else can explain the fact that innumerable songs, films, decorative items and books reflect our call and our search for love and happiness - basically the search for our true selves?
The longing for love, peace and harmony are signposts of our own expression. This longing becomes greater and more intense the more we experience the opposite in our lives. The more negativity, in other words, the more absence of that which we actually are and want, or presence of what we are not

and we do not want, the greater the longing for our own origin, eventually becoming a burning desire – a deep longing for something that simply does not leave us along, even if our mind wants to deny it.

The greatest longing or demand is for truly being oneself and experiencing and expressing oneself fully. Subconsciously we have recognized ourselves for a long time. We simply don't know what to do with this consciously, since the outer frame of reference and the consciousness of self-realization are missing.

Dreams and Wishes

The vague beginning of longing or desire are dreams that turn into wishes. Important wishes, which are not fulfilled for a long time, turn into longing and desire. Dreams are signposts that are trying to tell us something. According to current theories, some dreams serve simply to process experiences, the worst of these being nightmares. If also here we assume, that all is correct and important, we could conclude that dreams also have an entirely different meaning, about which we know nothing at this time.

However, there are dreams that point the way to our own longing and desires. Daydreaming or grand dreams or visions are not necessary desirable and were often criticized or even punished during our childhood. Various convictions that reduce dreams and hopes to a lesser value lay within each one of us. It is precisely those dreams and visions from our childhood that can show us the way back to ourselves. They are, figuratively speaking, a pointer to what our individual lives are about. When we are children, our connection to what we truly are, is still much deeper. We were still in touch with our true being and where we came from. There was just no one there who could teach us what to make of those dreams or of love and human relationships.

Big goals have one thing in common: they are always preceded by big dreams and hopes.

We know this quite well when it comes to our daily wishes, but not necessarily for the goals of the soul. The desire for peace in the world, peace and love in our surroundings, and within ourselves, are the reason why more and more people begin to develop their dreams, hopes and the soul's goal to create a new and different world, even if this appears to be utopian.

Hope

The flame of hope is important when apparent obstacles seem to block the way. Hope is the memory of the good that everyone carries within – at varying levels of visibility. In our times it is especially important, that we recognize and maintain our true goals to recognize and define a new path. This means, we need to say YES to new paths and goals and NO to the old ways. It is important that we fight our desire to "give up", that we face the challenges within and without, and that we learn to say NO to our own ways that do not serve us. This might possibly be the greatest challenge for each one of us, as well as collectively for all of us. It is important to properly question our self-doubt.

Václav Havel once said: *"Hope is not the conviction that something will turn out well but the certainty that something makes sense, regardless of how it turns out."*

This quote turns the „no" into the „yes". We turn the inner „yes" for our true self to take place instead of the outer „no" to our not serving world of success. We have forgotten the way to express our so often disowned self, that it seems to be like self-disowning when we say „No" to the outer circumstances of success which don't serve us. This „no" always renews the experience of this deeply hurting feeling of separation.

Conflict

To long for peace, recognition or love it requires a deficit: a conflict. Learning how to deal with conflicts is one thing; that there are good ways and less good ways is another. Desire or longing is actually present in order to initiate a thought process about what is wished for instead of the conflict. These thoughts can lead to self-empowerment and self-responsibility for doing everything in your power to create the conditions, where the conflict does not arise in the first place.

This is not about exchanging positive behavior for negative behavior, but rather about knowing what we REALLY WANT. Let us examine this using the example of the fear of death. Death is something we do NOT want. The focus is on DEATH. Thus automatically every thought and every action will be based upon what we do not want until now. If we change the focus and the definition to "fear of the loss of life", it automatically contains what we REALLY WANT, which is life. Now we have found the WHY behind the WHY and with it the original longing. Thus the longing can work for us and not against us. On that base we will realize much more details in our live, which don't serve us far beyond the topic of health itself. Now we are at that point, where we are able to realize all the things that don't serve the original goal of health in all that surrounds us. Now we become not only aware of the results of the rat race but we also become aware of the circumstances which led us to the rat race and all the causing situations with all its results. Therefore, a longing arises to change the original situations and what has led to the rat race, instead of only changing the results of the rat race. If we change our behavior which led us to the rat race, the whole circle of the negative rat race will switch into a positive flow-circle - the experience we are longing for. If we know this now, then we find it infinitely easier to apply the necessary action consistently, as we go to the true origin of our longing of change. A „towards-motivation" arises and replaces the „fromward-motivation". An unknown author once coined this wise quote: *"Know your WHY and start to FLY."* If we, as individuals or as a species, know what we really want, then, with the help of our longing, dreams will turn into desire to experience that, which has not yet been experienced.

Wishes

Wishes are more concrete than dreams and show where there may be potential in the individual areas of life and how to set clear goals. Longing has already grown, but the drive to action is not strong enough yet to prompt clear and concrete impulses for action. This wish is either not important enough yet, or it is considered to be impossible. The image of the wish is activated in the mind, but a clear goal that could be brought to life by similarly clear actions has not been defined. The focus is on problems connected with the wish situation, rather than on solution approaches.

Now we get to the core of today's challenges. Through the misunderstanding of ourselves and the resulting misunderstanding of success, we have blocked our own way to paradise on earth. The desire for peace, abundance and love seems to be in opposition to the desire for security, wealth and recognition. For our mind this enterprise seems to be impossible, because its orientation is toward survival, and it thinks that what we have created out there serves that purpose. If we now introduce the rat race into question, thus we question automatically ourselves and our survival, at least according to the interpretation of our so conditioned mind. The force that can turn the either-or situation into an as-well-as situation is our self-awareness, which can be found within that part of ourselves we have not really trusted in: our heart – the link and the connection to our true divinity.

Requirements for Change

Goals are an essential requirement for any change. Someone who does not really know what they want, will not be able to achieve effective change. In other words: *"If one does not know to which port one is sailing, no wind is favorable."* –Seneca

The great misunderstanding of ourselves and of success, along with all of its effects for the individual and for the collective, lets us see more clearly, why all the efforts on earth to resolve conflict in the best interests of all, were destined to fail. The real goal was never the focus, let alone known or admitted.

If the highest goal is to experience oneself as the best possible divine expression of peace, love, and part of divinity itself, the various concrete goals will appear in the individual areas of challenge and can then be turned into concrete actions via sub-goals. All actions are then in harmony with the overall goal.

Hold On

This is a very important point, in spite of all the talk about the importance of letting go. The question here is WHAT should be let go of and WHAT should be held onto.

It seems that we first must let go of various old convictions and the resulting thinking, feeling, words and actions. Anyone that believes in their wishes and dreams will be able to let go of quite a bit. Many people have simply not held on to what is REALLY important to them and have given up just before reaching the goal, because people with different convictions created doubt. This doubt is as reliable as the Amen in church, if we as humans want to make room for our common goal of self-awareness and the resulting logical consequences of collective-awareness and as result the wish to create „heaven on earth". The question is on the one hand whether we believe in it, and on the second hand, if we believe it long enough to do what's necessary and turn it into visible results.

The Power of Defeat

Every defeat contains the seed of a corresponding success. We shall use the following examples to demonstrate the power of the impossible:

Henry Ford was poor and uneducated, but he had a dream of a means of transportation that could work without draft animals. Did it all go well? NO, not at all! Were people enthusiastic about his plans in the beginning? NO, of course not! And yet, his unshakable drive and belief in his vision makes it possible for you and me to drive a car today. Our thanks should go to this man. Another example is Steve Jobs: He had the desire and the vision that every person should have a computer on his or her desk. At first people called him crazy, but he believed in it with a burning desire. Did it all go well? Of course not! Did he have setbacks and criticism? YES, of course, and plenty! Did he remain true to his dreams? YES, until they became reality! And today? You and I and many others all over the world have the machine on our desks that he dreamed of.

There are innumerable examples. Why shouldn't it be possible to make use of this for our health, our ideal love relationship, our relationship with ourselves, our family, the right career, or whatever? When dreams can come true, we may discover a much greater dream within us – the dream of our contribution to creating a positive new world, „heaven on earth". I don't consider this preposterous, but it's maybe about us to think of a totally new interpretation of what heaven looks like. I believe, that everyone has a dream that serves not only themselves, and I hope that everyone will find it at some point and hold on to it until it becomes reality. Will everything always go well? Probably not. Will there be criticism and setbacks, if we want to create „heaven on earth"? With absolute certainty! But what if, 50 years from now, our children and grandchildren are living in heaven on earth, and can look back and say: "Look at that... we can thank our parents and grandparents, and maybe great-grandparents for that". Dreams are the seeds of this world. Even the greatest achievement began with a dream!

The desire for change in this life, this burning desire and longing for real life and self-realization, is the starting point from which all dreams take to the sky. Dreams are not made of indifference, laziness/complacency or lack of action. Always remember, when you feel real low, full of doubt or you want to give up: all those who are successful in life, regardless in what area, have had to battle defeat sometime in their life. They had to go to battle before their dream could become reality.

Oftentimes the turning point is a moment of deep crisis, while becoming acquainted with our other self; a deeply painful experience, because we knew so little about it before. This other Self has been misunderstood.

The change has no need to be so painful as we experienced it before, because these misunderstandings caused the pains. If we as human beings come to understand ourselves, we come to the moment, where we replace pain by trust and hope and will see, that there is no such thing then pain but only misunderstandings. We will come to see, that just a piece of information or just a bigger awareness was amiss to realize the true gift and message of any situation. It seems as though humanity itself has now arrived at a memorable point of its deepest and greatest crisis. The potential for this turning point and our true BEING lay hidden within each of us and all of us at the same time.

Truth or Lies

In order to truly believe or trust in something, it may occasionally occur to us as if we were dealing with lies. When the mind is overloaded with negative limitations, searching for the positive counterpart with all its related content can seem like fantasy, sweet-talking or lies. Nevertheless, the counterpart exists at the same time and represents examining things from another point of view. If we evaluate things from the standpoint of the old truth, newly accepted thoughts will appear like lies, unless we make continuous updates to the complete truths, which includes uncovering old truths as misunderstandings. Eventually such updates show that the old truths now appear to be lies from the new point of view as well. It does not matter from which point of view truths are intermixed, because from the standpoint of conditional love they will always appear to be a lie. Only unconditional love will bring both parts together so that we can find out, that there was never a lie but multiple misunderstandings, because there is always just our own truth. There are at least two or more controversial perceptions. As the saying goes: *"We don't see the world the way it is, but how we are"* (A. Nin) When we recognize ourselves in love and as part of the divine, the biggest misunderstanding in the world can be resolved, and two or more opposing truths can still become as one, because they are no truths but only perceptions.

It is the assessment of a thing that determines the character of what we see. If we judge something positively the positive will appear, if we judge something negatively, the negative will appear.

There are two interesting experiments showing this:
Researchers compared test subjects who had arachnophobia with test subjects who did not. They used a stereoscope to show to one eye the picture of a spider, and the other eye a geometric form. The test subjects who had arachnophobia saw predominantly the spider, while the test subjects without the fear did not. It should be mentioned here that our eyes are capable of seeing only one object at a time, which means that fear will influence our perception. Both are present simultaneously,

the geometric form and the spider image, but the fear is what makes the difference.

A study was made where people who were considered lucky were to be compared to "unlucky" people. Test subjects were sought and chosen who saw themselves as lucky or unlucky. One after the other, the test subjects were sent to a café where the entrance had been prepared for the study; for this purpose, a five-pound note was placed at the entryway. Those who had signed up as the unlucky ones had all walked right past the bill, directly into the café. Those who considered themselves lucky found the bill. This shows that focus makes all the difference. The lucky people's perception is more open to the positive, while the unlucky ones' perception is closed in general, and to the positive in particular.

Our Future Is Up to Us

A very impressive example for truly big goals is the founder of Christianity. Jesus Christ was a prolific dreamer; he had a great deal of imagination. Ultimately his vision gave birth to Christianity, although his message unfortunately continued to be misunderstood. The pragmatic dreamers, and there have been many, have always been pioneers and architects of our civilization.
What works on such a large scale as religion must also work when many people remember and recall together, what the goal really is. If longing and desire, dreams, wishes and goals are in harmony with our true self, we can presume, that all of our actions are a compulsory thing that simply follows. Our only limitations are those of our thinking, which is based upon that, which has always been the way it was – a misunderstanding of our true self and with that, the misunderstanding of success.

"Perfection of means and confusion of ends seems to characterize our age." –Albert Einstein

2. Trust

Trust is indispensable and fundamental to success and is a determining factor for positive results.

What is behind the word "Trust"? It is related to confidence, which can easily be associated with courage. This courage increase when we are deeply connected with ourselves or to somebody. Therefore, self-confidence or self-trust is based upon one's own self-effectiveness. Under the influence of success and failure as we have defined it until now, only an incomplete image of self-confidence and self-trust is the result. Until now, success has been associated with action and money or property, and failure oftentimes with a lack of action and having little or no money or property. Actually our longing to DO NOTHING, or simply to BE, has the aim of bringing us into a space of peace and aloneness, so that we can become aware of our own misconceptions. But this would mean to our mind, by implication, that survival is no longer secure, because BEING is suddenly given higher priority. It takes courage to examine this misconception in detail.

The Beginning

Trust is inherent in all of us, and is our birthright. We have simply forgotten to trust ourselves and thus others. The first people we trust are our parents, or those who raise us. Depending upon how they dealt with us, we have developed lower or higher levels of trust. The number and type of reactions from our earlier environment determine, how much trust we develop – in ourselves, in people and in life. Actually, trust is not something that emerges from a person or circumstances outside of us. Rather, it originates in the connection with our inner self and is experienced externally as a resonance. It is the discrepancy between the self-perception and the external perception that first gives birth to a feeling of mistrust, creating fear and insecurity.

The more our original environment discredited our connection to ourselves through negative or fearful interventions, the more doubt arose in our self-confidence. Conversely, the external perception takes precedence over our self-perception, which means, that we give the statements and impulses from our environment more credence than our own inner impulses. Our own divine universal origin is then inevitably denied and forgotten. Physical dependency leads to the subconscious belief that those, who are already living on earth and care for us must know better, since they already have experience living in this world. Consequently, they should know how life works. Such a slew of misinterpretations could not be expected; they are all built upon the same misinterpretation of ourselves and love – and the lack of understanding of what true, unconditional love really is and what kind of success it aims to achieve.

Ralph Waldo Emerson, the American philosopher and writer, formulated this very appropriately: *"On the debris of our despair we build our character"*. This phrase illustrates what arises from the despair of being misunderstood as a "little person". We build our character from that which is left of our self-perception; this then shapes our individual lives.

Perception

Perception means to recognize something as truth. Truth, here, seems a bit like something static, while perception continues to be developing and appears to be malleable. Perception changes as soon as new information and realizations appear, which we were not aware of before - nevertheless they existed before.

Have you ever asked yourself what truth is? It seems as though we may have a misconception here as well; as though there were actually one single truth, but this truth is not connected to knowledge and action, but rather to the state of HOW. It seems that the only truth is LIVE AND LOVE, offering us an infinite number of opportunities for experiences and perceptions as an expression of the divine.

"The illiterates of the 21st century are not those who are unable to read and write, but those who do not learn, unlearn and relearn".
Alvin Toffler, the author and futurist, could not have said it more accurately. Our old truths make us illiterates of life. Only when we unlearn, question and examine those old truths, and acknowledge new truths in self-awareness and self-love, can we learn to read, understand and thus trust ourselves and life. The good news is that all of life is change -therefore even the illiteracy of the 21st century is subject to change.

Misunderstanding: Self-Confidence or Self-Trust

Even extremely strong and boisterous personalities may have little confidence inside; they are merely using their self-assured behavior to mask their old beliefs of deficiency or lack, since they have learned that they achieve better results that way. One might say they have found a reliable way to master life and survival such that more positive than negative remains in the end. They do not have the confidence that comes from trust in life, but believe that their own actions are the only things that one can and should trust. These people have learned to be successful based on conditional love. Often such people are in leadership positions in economics, politics or other institutions.

Through the contribution of all those in leadership positions who have confidently self-empowered themselves, our way of success leads to the worldview we are familiar with today. Teachers with a high level of self-awareness have taught us another worldview based on unconditional love, which seems to be diametrically opposed to the present system. As a consequence, this new worldview would inevitably confront the leaders of the present systems with their greatest pain and fear of loss – the fear of losing purpose and the accompanying fear of being alone. The meaning of life referred to here is linked to the same definition that is based on the misinterpretation of success, and this fear and the related pain are devastating. Thus this fear and pain are generally very well hidden and subconscious.

There is a creational process that we have so far used on the basis of conditional love in order to create what we see today. Heart and feeling show what we are able to accept as truth; they create a connection between feeling and intellect. The subconscious becomes active on the basis of our belief in the definition of success. Feelings of trust are restored. The mind begins to forge concrete plans to attain the desired goal. Unconditional love uses exactly the same creational process. We would be able to create something like holistic success, by using the best of our current success-model and by expanding it with true self-awareness as a divine being and true self-confidence. The best possible result for all involved would become possible. Every step along this path – no matter how small – strengthens the cycle of trust if we give heed to our inner voice and inner impulses.

Misunderstanding Self-Awareness

What we call self-awareness or self-assurance is actually based upon a slight misinterpretation that has serious consequences.

The word "self-awareness" expresses nothing more than being certain or aware of our (own) self. Our interpretation of self-awareness is based on our success until now, and consists of knowing one's own positive and negative patterns of thinking and behavior, feelings and speech, and applying them in a positive, successful manner within our current context of success. It is not based upon the notion that we know and experience ourselves to be divine universal beings. Our interpretation has been limited to the external consequences, e.g. our self-confident behavior, which is really only self-assured behavior. True self-assurance has nothing to do with how strong someone appears outwardly. There is no indication with regard to dominance. Until now, that which we call self-awareness or self-assurance has been based upon conditional love.

It might be good that many more people are much more consciously aware of themselves and their divine core than they think they are, and are outwardly not seen as self-assured according to the old interpretation. However, our erroneous definition of success leads to a misinterpretation of their self-confidence, which means that these people will not live out the unconditional love inherently present within them, because they either do not trust in their inner voice, or their external circumstances make living this love seemingly impossible. Self-awareness without the necessary self-confidence will do little; it may even lead to the opposite effect, resulting in massive self-condemnation, since they are consciously aware that so much is recognized and known about oneself and universal laws without being able to implement success-promoting changes. The external context is not in alignment with the inner realizations.

Turbo Jet to the Core of Our Trust

The conditions we call trust, love and sexuality are very powerful in their own right. Combined, the three of them can connect us directly to our core. When they trigger brain impulses together they are much more powerful than any of them individually; even more so if conditional love becomes unconditional love through true awareness.
Trust is also fostered when these three aspects come together based upon the old way of thinking, however this old, conditional love is actually based on fear.
It is irrelevant which brain impulse is triggered by trust, the subconscious will translate the impulse according to our belief and our level of trust. This is why we still all too often end up with

non-satisfactory results in many situations, although we try to the best of our ability to achieve a favorable outcome. This happens because our current turbo tandem still consists of trust, sexuality and fear, disguised as that which we have learned to perceive as love. Our deep-rooted desire for a partner relationship subconsciously wants to show us, that a part of our soul knows the original laws, but they have been misinterpreted and thus are not "properly" integrated into our lives. This part of us knows, that our love relationships and partnerships, as well as trust and sexuality we have experienced thus far, are capable of bringing forth an entirely new and different result on all levels, in combination with unconditional love. Subconsciously, love relationships make us naturally more courageous and stronger, and make us more aware of the trust in ourselves and others. We will discuss the subject of love, sexuality and their meanings and consequences in more detail in the last chapter of this book, as they would exceed the scope of this chapter.

Built on Sand

The fact remains, that our subconscious will just as readily produce malicious and negative thoughts as it will positive ones. It all depends on which environment has influenced us the most in life. If we want to build trust, we should ask ourselves on what basis we build our trust. Whom or what we trust externally, shows the measure of, or the discrepancy with our internal self-trust.

Let's compare this with a wheat kernel: the seed is sown and falls on fertile ground, is watered and tended to. It sprouts into a plant that bears fruit in much greater numbers than originally. Once sown and cultivated, the grain bears fruit. This grain of wheat is like our thoughts that are based on our trust, which stems from that which we consider truth. Whether we sow positive or negative thoughts, we will reap what we sow. The seeds sown multiply with each sowing and harvest. The fruits of the harvest will depend on which thoughts are the most present.

This "wheat example" demonstrates, how the proportions can be mixed anew, again and again, depending upon which thought-seeds we given preference to. Every thought, plan, goal and intention is followed by a multitude of similar thoughts, and combines these energies and powers, so that a consonance can be formed of the similar thoughts and energies. This consonance will eventually grow into the main stem; this is simply caused by repetition. Any given thought or intention can take hold in the mind by way of repetition. Seen over the course of a lifetime, it becomes clear why there is such a thing as "good luck" or "bad luck".

The Why

The entire universe revolves around the "why". Is the "why" of our daily actions love or fear? The results could not be any different. The following saying from the Talmud demonstrates this very well:

"Watch yourself.
 Watch your words, for they become deeds.
 Watch your deeds, for they become habits.
 Watch your habits, for they become your character.
 Watch your character, for it becomes your destiny."

Today's reality is the result of our seeds – those things that we have sown based on our beliefs about success. We have trusted in this path for a very long time, although we may wonder again and again, why so much violence and cruelty are present in this world – on both the large and small scale. We still have not understood that the small is much more related to the large than we would think – which is why it has been said for some time: changing yourself from the inside is the solution. This is certainly a large portion of the truth, but not the whole truth. At a certain point change is also required in the environment otherwise the flow will be interrupted.

A Strong Vision

According to various studies, it takes approximately 21 days of regular practice to form a habit. Then the first plateau is reached and it becomes easier and easier. After about 6 months the new behavior has become second nature.

Let's take a moment to imagine what would be possible, if we could establish new trust in ourselves and our experience of love and success, and how new habits could develop from that. If enough people would be willing to experience love and success in a different way for just 6 months, the world would have the chance to change significantly. Would that not be worth a try, even for those who don't really believe in it? If it works, we all win, and if it doesn't, we would not have lost anything worth mentioning.
We recognize this principle on the basis of the outstanding example of Gandhi. He created a situation in which trust in a very specific goal grew in the hearts and minds of millions of people. By these means, he accomplished what no military power has ever achieved – without money, soldiers or weapons of war. He caused all of those people to unite and to act in harmony as though they were of one mind and spirit – which is indeed the case. What would be possible if we all work together, a few more each day, to create paradise on earth? Actually it appears that an increasing number of us are doing this already.
Let us develop a truly wonderful idea of the life we would like to live. Let us trust that we deserve it and that it comes from within us. Then we call this idea to life with the help of our imagination. We break the big picture, the vision, the dreams and goals down into smaller pictures, which are our sub-goals. Let's develop actionable plans for each one of these sub-goals. If our sub-goals are too large, we break them down into sub-sub-goals. Then we carry out our implementation with perseverance and work toward completion with unconditional determination. Our burning desire for peace, health and love on this

earth, and in our own life experience as it is anchored within us as an idea, will smooth the way there.

Trust is the elixir that breathes life into all of our pursuits, awakening power and effectiveness in our thoughts.

3. Inner Dialogue and Autosuggestion

The way we talk to ourselves determines our success, whether by our old or new definition, no matter what. Autosuggestion is the power of our thinking and the means by which the subconscious mind is influenced. Autosuggestion is the dialogue each one of us carries out with ourselves, consciously or subconsciously, in words or in thoughts. According to Wikipedia, the definition of autosuggestion is as follows: *"auto-suggestion (Greek/Latin: auto-influence) is the process by which a person trains his or her subconscious mind to install a belief. This can be attained through self-hypnosis or repeated self-affirmations and can be considered a form of self-induced influence on the psyche. The effectiveness of auto-suggestive thought formulations can be enhanced by mental visualization of the desired goal. The success of practicing autosuggestion becomes more likely with consistent and prolonged (or more frequent) use…"*

The thoughts and visualized goals we allow to play an essential role in our lives – positive or negative, conscious or subconscious – all serve this principle and result in creating our reality. Autosuggestion originates through suggestions from outside. Meditation is suggestion. Education is suggestion. The continuous stream of information from the media is suggestion. If repeated enough, anything imaginable can be suggestion and can become autosuggestion. Another term for this is dogmas or belief-systems – those thoughts we have and statements we make based on our internal truth. Parents, religion, society, the economic system, politics and media are the backbones of our autosuggestions.

Three Great Mantras of Our Time

Our erroneous definition of success has brought us to allow the following phrases to create our daily reality (truth), consciously or subconsciously: "I don't have enough time", "I don't have enough money" and "I don't have the connections or relationships". These 3 sentences bear out the entirety of our fundamental misunderstandings.

"I don't have enough time" cannot be accurate, as everyone has exactly the same 24 hours a day. The real question we humans should ask ourselves is this: For whom or for what do we use the 24 hours of life time each day?

"I don't have enough money" is also a misconception, considering how well-off we are in comparison to many other regions in the world. It appears instead, that our interpretation of success has led us to believe, that money and the resulting means and goods and their related consumption, have been assigned a value that is not healthy for us. This leaves the question: for whom or for what is this money being used?

Finally, the statement, "I don't have the relationships" seems to be the most impactful, as it shows what our misconception of success really entails. Our current definition of success says that we would be more successful if only we maintained the right connections or relationships. In our pursuit of riches, we frequently lose the connection to our inner self and to the most important people and values along our way – only to be replaced by our relationship to a career, a job, and the corresponding environment. The value of our connections is subconsciously measured by what material benefits these may provide. According to the wording of this statement, relationships that appear to provide no material benefits are of absolutely no value. It is hardly surprising then, that we invest our time primarily where material gains appear to be likely and therefore lose sooner or later these relationships, which are important for our true longing and desire for love, health and peace. This is not only about the relationship and connection between human beings but also about all things, situations and circumstances. So we should ask ourselves: With whom or with what do we keep our most intensive relationships? Do we nurture our relationships to things more than those to ourselves, other people or nature?

If we were to redefine our notion of success and place love at the core of our definition, those 3 sentences would be obsolete and simply invalid. As long as we pay tribute to our current definition of success, these phrases will be the autosuggestion to many of us, who will continue to ask, why so many things seem to be wrong in life and on earth.

The Counterpart

Let's turn from education, politics and religion to those answers we have given ourselves for quite some time without being aware of them. In songs, novels, poetry, decorative items, postcards, books of wisdom and films, and in many other forms, love is still at the center – interestingly enough, even our numerous action films and thrillers seem to always touch on the topic of love. This is one way that our subconscious yearning for our origin manifests itself. Suggestions regarding creative work appear like the souls calling to itself and, through our feelings, create a yearning as well as other thoughts and autosuggestions that stand in opposition to the daily grind of our self-created "success hamster wheel", with all its obligations and responsibilities. Through our positive feelings we begin to resonate with these wonderful messages that are intended to wake us up, thus creating increasingly more moments of self-awareness, even though we may not be aware of it at the time.

The Leading Role

Our spirit and mind accept only the thoughts that are permeated by feelings and emotions to translate into success. This is success factor no. 1 for change, regardless in which direction.

Thoughts with negative emotions will also become reality, just as thoughts with positive emotions will. The moment we infuse feelings and emotions into these thoughts, something comes to life in us. Feelings are an expression of the soul, signaling harmony with one's personal truth through the positive and disharmony with one's personal truth through the negative. Positive and negative feelings are living expressions; this enthusiasm is our expression.

With this in mind, it is hardly surprising that we need these "creations of love and wisdom" to become increasingly prominent in word, text, song and film. They create a balance to the constantly increasing negative messages and horror scenarios, and point the way to our natural desire for self-expression through love.

Control

We humans were created to have control over that which penetrates our subconscious and that which doesn't. Most people make little or no use of this, since they are simply unaware of it or have no knowledge of it. One simple method of controlling and disciplining oneself in the area of negative feelings is, to limit the amount of fear-mongering media and people as much as possible. This enables us to use this space instead for our own development of things and people that are more positive and conducive to our growth. It is up to us whether we want to be continuously kept up-to-date on the horror stories in this world, thereby exacerbating our experience of fear, or if we want to turn to the positive messages that also exist, but which are not quite as easily accessible. We ourselves decide what type of music we hear on a continual basis. We ourselves determine what types of people and their "music" we want to be predominantly exposed to.

Let's switch from external to internal "music". The paragraph above certainly does not mean that we should have absolutely no interest in what goes on in the world. In fact, it seems imperative that we realize and take seriously many things inside of a much larger overall context. The point is to recognize that fear will not support us if we really want to impact any of our challenges. At this juncture it is important to recognize that our own inner selves can learn to deal with this, and to step out of the entanglements and misinterpretations of what we call success. We are called upon to turn away from the noise and fear outside, to face the own inwards, so that we learn to understand us and therefore, what is happening around us. The connection to love, the source of original power and wisdom within us, shows us ways to deal with and to change these challenges; they can doubtless be resolved from a state of love but this would be in a completely different way as what we are used to know.

One simple method of making the soul's desire more tangible and to express it, is to set it out in writing. Thus the longing is brought from energetic, thought-based manifestation into the corresponding physical, material realm.

Another way to strengthen positivity in ourselves is to use autosuggestion exercises, spoken aloud every morning and evening. Particularly in times of numerous fearful scenarios, strengthening one's self from the inside is of great significance before changing something outside.

Feedback

Positive and negative feedback can be interpreted as suggestion from an external source. This is why it is so important to give positive feedback. To speak one's own truth is very important, however, the words we use should be chosen thoughtfully and in peace. The more we are able to formulate things we don't like in a positive manner, the more we strengthen each other, and the more inner strength, self-confidence and self-reliance will grow, because we are reminded of who we really are. This is how we can support each other by not being occupied with or burdened by the omnipresent crisis scenarios. Instead, we can support each other by reaching a state of inner strength that can make solutions to the scenarios possible. One autosuggestion exercise that can help to master internal and external challenges is to ask: *"What would love do now?"*

Anyone that knows what is wanted instead, will sooner or later find the means and ways to avoid "conflict situations" to begin with. There is the awareness, that previously another reality, and therefore another situation, can be conceived and can hence be created. For this new reality, completely different ways of thinking, feeling, speaking and acting will be adopted.

Concentration

Concentration refers to a targeted focus on a specific thing. WHAT WOULD BE THE COMMON SPECIFIC THING, if success would no longer be the core point and split into poor and rich, powerful and helpless, outspoken and silent, overeating and starving and small and large, but would be instead based upon the divine energy of love and connectedness?

If we really intend to change our lives, individually as well as globally – and both are inseparably connected – we will not be able to avoid making use of the tool of concentration.

Many philosophers have said, that man is the creator of his own destiny – and they are right! Each individual and all together, we are the masters of our destiny. If we once again make the power and responsibility of love our own, we have the chance to steer our destiny in a positive direction. It is our job to be our own „Father and Mother God", in ways our parents were not able to be, because they did not know the truths and laws of true love, divinity and success; they were not aware of their true selves. On this path we not only have the chance to transform our lives into the lives we always wanted – we can also bring about atonement and healing of old wounds. If we can muster up the courage and the strength to face ourselves and our fears, each one of us will find peace within and carry this peace into the world.

Let us not wait for the perfect plan. Let us rather begin to change ourselves and the world, and expect and demand of our subconscious, that it reveals to us the respective plans or action steps. "The journey IS the destination" is the maxim that will keep us moving forward.

4. Observation, Personal Experience and Knowledge

Experiences, knowledge and the gift of observation are important prerequisites for any kind of success. If we look at our education system, we can see that schools, universities and other educational institutions distribute pretty much all the knowledge our present times have to offer. Regardless of how extensive or multifaceted this knowledge may be, however, it does not seem to contribute significantly to reaching our goals of true love, peace and healthy coexistence.

Knowledge is power! Is that really true? It might be more accurate to say, that knowledge is potential power!
Anyone that expresses wishes and desires through targeted actions will be able to enjoy the experience of knowledge as power. Unfortunately, our current type of success has produced what we have experienced as power throughout the millennia and what we continue to experience today. It seems that we are lacking a proper goal-directedness, independent of the results, which makes all of our knowledge useless in terms of fulfilling our deepest longing for true love, health and peace. Apparently our current way of goal setting does not seem to be adequate.

The lack of understanding regarding goal setting is the reason that every day millions of people stumble over the erroneous belief that "knowledge is power" and wonder why they get "B" when they wanted "A". This misunderstanding is based upon the observations and experiences through external knowledge like our own experiences, school knowledge, knowledge through training, research-based knowledge, societal knowledge, etc. In the perpetual comparison between outer and inner knowledge, so to speak knowledge of our divine-spiritual origin, potentials and responsibilities, these realms seem to be diametrically opposed to each other. The effects of these two realms impair the power over our own self, life and all correlated circumstances.

Effects

It is a common assumption that someone is referred to as educated, if they have a great deal of general and special knowledge. However, the world is full of such educated people who are nonetheless not particularly successful and are not at all happy. Observations and experiences of each individual and of all of us create a bizarre image of us as human beings.
This large amount of general and specialized knowledge does not seem capable of empowering us to create that, which seems to be the most important to us all: peace, health and a loving and respectful coexistence.

We use this ever-increasing specialized knowledge to create ever-newer and more creative things, that are intended to make our daily lives easier and more enjoyable, so that we finally have time to be happy. More and more new computer games are created, which allow us to ascend to ever-higher levels by mastering the challenges of the game. More toys are invented that communicate interactively with children, sometimes replacing real animals or even us as their playmates. Ever-newer food fabrications are invented and manufactured, as is the case with decorative items and practical tools for our daily routing. Creativity seems to know no boundaries in every sector of our lives, yet it is not capable of providing us inner and outer peace or harmony.

It seems that the time has come to invest all of this creativity in a much larger goal, so that instead of the fictional computer world, new levels can finally be reached in the real world to get a New World. Maybe it's time, instead of ever-newer creations of delicious and visually pleasing foods, to prevent several hundred people from starving to death each hour, while we are thinking about how to refine and beautify this or that dish. In spite of the sum total of all of our knowledge and all of our experiences, we have not yet managed to create conditions that can be called humane for all of us. How can this be?

One possible and somehow logical answer might be, that we are forging ahead on the wrong side of development. We explore to the smallest, how detailed various processes in plants, animals, humans, the environment and the universe are working, all the while overlooking a great commonality: all of these processes function AUTOMATICALLY. Neither plants, nor animals, nor the environment, nor the universe must be taught how to create growth and continued development as a natural success. Could it be, that with all of this research of the HOW, we are overlooking the THAT of natural automatism, not realizing, that all of our external efforts to create automation out in our lives - over millennia and particularly in the past 100 years - are basically a reflection of our merely never understood automation of the divine universal energy within us, manifested as the ethics of our soul, because we are perpetually standing in its way with great determination and at times even violence? No other species behaves this way. No other species destroys and deprives itself of its own basis of existence the way we human beings do. Success, as we have learned to interpret it, stands above self-love and the love of others.
It seems possible, that if we invite love with all of their consequences into our lives, we will automatically experience HOW everything functions, and that it then all seems totally logical, because we see ourselves as part of the whole and therefore know, that we will also create increasingly higher levels of success from within and through our actions. It is time to invite our true humanity – we will still be successful, only on a much more satisfying and truly fundamental and life-affirming basis. If we

choose to, we can recognize, that our attempts at the automation of our environment and external things are based on the desire to HAVE more, so that we someday will have enough time and money to take care of BEING that human being we want to be. Here again we can recognize that this process is backwards – not wrong, but in the wrong order. The original context of BE-DO-HAVE has been misunderstood and turned into DO-HAVE-BE. When we recognize that we could all act according to the same divine universal conditions, we will see that BEing is not something we need to become, but rather something we have long since been and have merely forgotten. When we begin DOing according to that, which emerges from this self-realization, we will HAVE success across every board. And the process will reverse then.

By the Beard of the Prophet

A truly educated and wise human being is someone whose mind/spirit is developed the way, that all desires are fulfilled without infringing on the rights of others. Outer and inner knowledge are in harmony in body, mind and spirit, and are unified into wisdom. Action is aimed at the best possible results for all involved. This happens automatically, when self-love and self-realization are at the center of Being, Doing and Having. Yes, it happens automatically, because it is a profound spiritual need and corresponds to the ethics of our soul.
One very important word must be pointed out here: Will. Success, as we know it, brings forth another kind of will than the success that is based upon unconditional love. We have forgotten what we really want. Dreams, goals and visions that were in harmony with our true origin were repressed, bit by bit, by the framework of success as we are used to. Until now it seems impossible, that the heart's true longing could ever be fulfilled. Here we once again encounter those three phrases again: "I don't have the money, I don't have the time, and I don't have the connections". At his point in our personal life and the point

which human history faces today, we will have no choice but to examine these three sentences more closely:

1. Little or no money: Here we need to ask: Who has the money? Who has how much money? What is it being used for? Does it serve the healing, the sustained support and the wellbeing of each individual and the whole surrounding world, or does it serve the unconscious, or sometimes conscious destruction of our own bodies, other people or the surrounding world?

2. No time: For whom or for what do we use the 24 hours of life time each day? Do they serve the healing, the sustained support and wellbeing of each individual's relationship with himself, the relationships with all of the surrounding world, or do they serve the unconscious, or sometimes conscious destruction of our own bodies, other people and the surrounding?

3. No relationships: With whom or with what do we keep our most intensive relationships? Do we nurture our relationships to things more than those to ourselves, other people or nature? Do these relationships serve to support our expression of ourselves and the healing of our self, our surroundings and the world surrounding us? Or do these relationships serve, unconsciously or sometimes consciously, to deny or destroy our own self, other people, our surrounding or the surrounding world?

A Worthy Purpose

This is a very important point: a worthy purpose, the meaning, the WHY! All of the knowledge that we collect, adopt or experience, only makes any REAL SENSE, when it is in the context of our true human origin, our divinity. The life's work of each individual and of humanity is then fully usable. Our life's work is a result of the aspects of our lives that are relevant and important to each individually. A part within us has an idea of what is important to us, knows our life's work, and tries to lead us through gut feeling and intuition, so that we will do those things that are important to achieve this. Our daily routine, which is based on our current interpretation of success, all too often involves, that we act against this feeling in favor of social standards – and in constant betrayal of ourselves. This betrayal is, what leaves us dissatisfied and unhappy, since our actions do not reflect what makes sense to our soul, because they are opposed to and are not aligned with our actual purpose. Our knowledge has the usefulness we are longing for when we empower it with its worthy purpose and the connection of our true origin.

Ambition – an Underestimated Accomplice

One human weakness, for which there seems to be no remedy, is the lack of ambition.
According to the dictionary, ambition means *"vigorous strive for"*. As happens so often, it has been interpreted in a negative way. Only in more recent times did we find a definition for so-called positive ambition.
If we proceed on the premise that each individual soul on this earth has the one goal of realizing itself, then this *"vigorous striving for"* gets an entirely new meaning. From this point of view, it is only too natural to conclude, that ambition is an essential ingredient for finding oneself or becoming self-aware. Here again misinterpretation leads us astray and creates a definition of ambition for success as we know it, with all of its undesirable consequences.
Given our lack of knowledge of our own destiny and the ensuing misjudgment of fear, this could only result in a misinterpretation of the word. As a logical consequence, a negative anchoring of the word "self-awareness" follows. This definition often leads to a disdain of people who appear self-confident, their behavior being misunderstood as arrogance, which, as we know, comes before the fall. A part of our humanity seems to sense intuitively, that this expression is not accurate in its original meaning, since unconditional love seems to be absent and

therefore the actions are not in harmony with the true root of self-confidence and self-awareness. The question is, what falls? Until now this question has always come from the perspective of fear. As a result, a part of us always experiences doubt, because there is a kind of discrepancy in the definition of our values. Ambition yes, ambition no, self-confidence yes, self-confidence no – but always in just the right measure, please. And just what is this measure? A sense of struggle and high caution, as well as a fear of certain failure arise with these questions. Let's try another approach.
Could it be that it is old limitations and convictions that fall here, as soon as courage - instead of pride - ambition and true self-awareness enter the room? When these characteristics are seen from the perspective of unconditional divine love, the source of our soul, they actually become meaningful.

Life is a perpetual process of change – a process of acquiring knowledge, learning, unlearning, and re-learning again, which is, if examined closer, just a remembering. The POWER OF HABIT requires ambition based on the new definition of love; this provides considerable support in breaking old habits in favor of new ones, so that the deep yearning for inner and outer peace, inner and outer love and inner and outer health, that seems to slumber within so many of us, can be fulfilled – the most worthwhile goal mankind can have.

Ambition can also be analyzed in an entirely different manner. Our current path led to a situation in which we have the highest regard for those, who achieve the greatest musical, theatrical, sports or financial performances etc. All other categories are given far less recognition. Honors are granted those, who have succeeded in acquiring vast amounts of money. One logical consequence of unconditional divine love could be, to curb the recognition and approval for those things, that we until now have defined as the greatest successes in the world, or to recognize that great success in sports, theatre, voice and finance, has the same value, that the success of development aid workers, tutors, teachers, social workers, or parents have. No matter how we look at it, it is time for a more appropriate definition in the sense of true equality, in other words a state of „the same true value", instead of indifference, which would put an end to the sense of indifference (as in apathy) that does not serve us.

The Opportunity

The fact that life and our own role are constantly subject to change is based upon perception. With each new piece of knowledge, with each expansion of our perception, it is possible that old truths change and are no longer tenable. Life is suddenly quite different than it seemed to be when we add new insights. With each additional expansion of our perception and each acquisition of special knowledge, there is an opportunity to arrive at a new truth. At first this may sound exhausting, but this process invites us to find our way back to our origin. Until now we have all too often fought the acceptance of that, which is simply natural – it is this fight, that makes it seem so exhausting.

Actually, nothing new needs to be learned. Insights and truths have been there all along – they have simply not been perceived, and definitely not taken seriously, for a very long time. That part of us that is connected to everything, remembers how it was all meant to be before we allowed life to superimpose impressions and patterns. At the moment of remembering our original truth a very unique feeling arises. It is a flash of insight and deep knowledge, that it all now makes sense. Ease, joy and exhilaration arise with this. There is a profound certainty that "you know that you know" – a feeling of having arrived home. Sometimes this is accompanied by tears of relief and insight, and sometimes by tears of pain because we realize suddenly all these parts of life, having not lived since now.

The Power of an Idea

Behind every desire for change is an idea: The idea that there must be another or a better way. At times it seems bizarre, that we humans apply special knowledge to research the universe in order to make the idea of life or survival out there possible - life under unfavorable conditions - while at the same time destroying our paradise here on earth bit by bit. We seem to forebode, that we will not be able to survive on our own planet much longer, if we continue this way.

Special knowledge is, so to speak, the birthplace of new ideas. Unfortunately, most people have access to a great deal of special knowledge, but too little inner and outer access to soul ethics and the resulting ideas of how this knowledge may be applied to the current situations in the most sensible and, above all, the most expedient way.

Ideas and visions could contribute to the possibility of creating solution approaches for all areas of life through imagination and fantasy. Recognizing the positive habit behind a negative habit, and therefore recognizing the real goal, each individual contributes to the fact, that ideas and solution approaches can be provided for the current challenges on our planet.

People Helping People

More and more people feel that "something big" is waiting inside of them and embark on a path to find their "why". The number of people who want to work as a coach increases daily. These people seem to have recognized that their own path to self-awareness and self-expression has revealed opportunities and solutions, that may serve others. These people have recognized their own potentials, which – in these challenging times – serve to heal old injuries and misinterpretations, so that more and more people's true potentials and life work can come to light. They help to make visible the ideas and action steps necessary to overcome the challenges. One reason this professional group is experiencing such a boom seems to be, that as many people as possible can be guided to self-awareness as quickly as possible. The potentials, knowledge and ideas that are necessary to collectively master the challenges we have collectively created, lay slumbering in each of us who follows this consciousness. Accurately spoken, we need to know HOW this knowledge and all our achievements can be used, which are already here right now, in order to use them for the goals of unconditional love, unconditional health and unconditional peace.

Very Special Knowledge

For quite some time our planet has been steadily exploited. The impactful and destructive consequences could not be seen or recognized at first. Meanwhile, however, scientists have recognized, that the consequences of what has taken place successively over the years, could increase exponentially. If man does not make considerable changes, the predicted scenarios may well occur, and only too soon. Exponential growth is the word of the hour here.
Anyone interested in learning more about this can obtain more detailed information on the Internet at HYPERLINK http://www.peakprosperity.com/crashcourse/.

We may well be running out of time. Findings seems to substantiate, that the development of exponential growth has entered the final phase. Everything that went on for decades with barely any visible consequences will suddenly begin to experience rapid changes in ever-shorter periods of time – that is the nature of exponentiality.
But this principle works not only for negative development but equally for positive development. This principle even brings an opportunity for us to reverse this exponentially negative curve

under the influence of unconditional love, self-awareness and self-realization as a stepping stone to reverse the effects. Then the worst possible scenario would not occur and the best possible scenario would be possible. One could even say, that we are only one decision away from paradise.

Compare this to the life stories for example of Neale Donald Walsch, Eckhart Tolle, Wayne Dyer or even older examples such as Saulus who became Paulus. At the turning point of massive destruction or self-destruction they woke up and made serious changes to their reality and its expression. What may be possible, when at the point of most severe self-destruction humankind awakens and changes its expression completely?
Our human past and all related experiences and developments make sense only, when we no longer forget or deny our soul's origin, but rather remember, acknowledge and integrate it and, above all, act accordingly.

5. Intellect and Understanding

When we look at our general and specialized knowledge we might assume, that we have a pretty good intellect (= the faculty of reasoning and understanding objectively). However, when we look at the consequences of our actions and the conditions of many people and this world we can see, that there must be something we have not understood.

Comparison of information requires a keen intellect and a clear mind. But what do "keen intellect" and "clear mind" actually mean?
Negative and positive emotions cause us to awaken from our deep slumber, especially when they appear alternately and with high intensity. If we focus on a clear mind we can see, that it is not about our intellect, but rather the divine mind or spirit in each one of us, which is often not clearly visible, or even denied.

The following quote of R. Niebuhr speaks to the challenges that face mankind: *"God, grant me the serenity to accept the things I cannot change, courage to change the things I can, and the wisdom to know the difference."* Until now, this quote has largely been interpreted in such a way, that the circumstances on this earth are things we cannot change and that it would be wise to never question this, so that our inner peace and serenity will not be lost, or may at least be found again. Interestingly enough, this image actually contributes to the belief, that nothing on earth can really change for the better, since this judgment is based upon fear and conditional love with its corresponding view of success. What if it is the other way around?

When we look at this misunderstanding in an awakened state of awareness of our true origin, the phrase above can also be interpreted very differently. *"God, give me the serenity to accept my divine origin, which I cannot change, the courage to change the things in myself and in the world which I can change, and the wisdom to know the difference".*

Here, the first part of this phrase is an expression of our knowledge of our true origin and potential. We may twist and turn any way we want, the divine origin in everything does not disappear simply because we refuse to acknowledge it. The second part of the sentence refers to the responsibility for us ourselves and all that surrounds us. The third part refers to fact, that it seems not to be easy to know the difference, unless you are really aware who you truly are.

The Path

We have learned to consider things that are unexplainable or cannot be proven to be non-existent – an approach that, thank God, is progressively changing. The unconditional love, we brought with us at birth, is something that can neither be explained nor proven. It was not acknowledged; therefore, it does not exist, according to our brain and our definition. Life could not be UNDERSTOOD based on the original context, because the respective resonance was absent due to the lack of knowledge of it in the environment.

Children are inherently blessed with the three main components of love, trust and imagination. However, this was largely dispelled through upbringing by adults who also had this dispelled by their adults, who also had this dispelled by their adults ... and so on. We have forgotten what it is to see, feel and perceive based upon unconditional love, which is why success automatically turned into something else. Yet every generation has realized a bit more than the generation before, and we attempt to this day, to become the next best version of that, who we already are.

If You Don't Turn Out Like the Children

What we ourselves have learned, we impose upon our children like blinders – as the final word. Children are mostly considered to be innocent – divine – small beings whom, we simply seem not to understand. Who says that children don't see more than we adults do? Is it possible that from birth on they try to remind us of who we really are, simply by their existence? At this point I would like to refer to the chapter on autosuggestion, or rather the suggestions, which we have all heard ad nauseam and which have left their deepest impressions: "You're too young for that", "You don't understand that yet", "Won't you stop asking why". The most common question from children is "why", so I ask us: why? Could it be that our children, as soon as they are able to speak, are asking this question, because they want to understand the discrepancy between their inner truth and the external, practiced truth? Could it not be, that by repeatedly asking "why", they hope to bring us to question, what we say and do so self-evidently, often ourselves blind to the discrepancies in regard to our own true self and the true values inside? Yet how often do we respond with anger, lack of understanding or even fury, because we first of all have no time for an adequate answer, and secondly because true questioning gives rise to uncomfortable feelings such as powerlessness and lack of understanding on our end, with all of its consequences. Isn't it obvious that our children are here to remind us of our own misunderstood child within? Is maybe healing found less in all of the injuries and hurts but more in the wonderful and divine potentials we carry within us, which went misunderstood by misunderstanding unconditional love and therefore success, as they were originally intended. Isn't it true, that our children often suffer from the same misunderstandings we experienced in our childhood, although the manifestations can also be so opposite? As children we also tried in vain to convey this divine message to our parents. Conditions have been what they are for an infinite long time, because a misunderstanding at the root of everything results in a cascade of impressions of what life seems to be. This way of learning life seems to oppose the divine universal order in many respects.

An Important Role

Our brain is the transmitting and receiving station for our thoughts. Thoughts gain relevance and effect when they are mixed with emotions – this is how we breathe life into them. Metaphorically speaking, emotions are our color filters that color our reality. When in love, we speak of pink glasses, when depressed everything is seen in grey. All emotions stem in the duality of the emotions of fear and love; the brain translates what we present it. It constantly compares inner and outer truths. Negative emotions indicate, that something is not in harmony with the inner truth of "who I really am". Everything we built upon one big misunderstanding will point the way toward true understanding. With all of our technology and progress, we have come to the point where many people experience deep fears and an overwhelming feeling of aloneness in the misunderstood context. If all is one and all is love, then we can realize, that a big chance could wait within here. We are at a point, where severe fears can be transformed into love and where these deep feelings of aloneness can be transformed into oneness - just by awareness and therefore understanding.

The Marvel in Our Head

We still know relatively little about the power of our thoughts. However, it is becoming increasingly clear, that our thoughts together with our emotions, are the authors of our reality. Bit by bit, more light is shed on this mystery. Neuroscience is still in its infancy, but what has emerged so far is, that the brain has considerably more significance than previously assumed. Meanwhile it is obvious, that the cerebral cortex serves much more than merely physical growth and life-sustaining functions.

The cerebral cortex is designed like a highly differentiated communication network. This gives rise to the justified question as to whether the brain was primarily designed for communications at a higher level, with powers that are as yet unattainable and not understandable.

Such a masterpiece might well serve the purpose to communicate and interact in completely different ways with itself and the world, then it has until now. This masterpiece has the capacity to communicate not only with other human beings, but it also seems to be an interface for communication with everything in existence. Therefore, it should be no surprise, that such a very small percentage of the brain has been actively used to date. Maybe this is because we did not know how to use it adequately and sensibly. Until now we did not have the perception. For perceiving something as really true, it may require a new, different emotion: the emotion of unconditional love, divine energy itself, since this entails the realization that everything originates from the same energy, and that therefore so much more is possible than we have ever thought. Consequently, this implies that communication should be possible with everything in existence. Moreover, it also means that ultimately, through this connection to all that exists, we also carry the responsibility for all that exists.

Invisible Forces

They are something that more and more people believe in, simply because they have experiences that cannot be explained from a human perspective, or with numbers, data or facts.
We are at the cusp of a new age, where a larger and more powerful picture of our own true self and all of the resources and potentials connected to it emerges. It is an era in which the divine essence becomes visible and intellect or mind can, slowly but surely, be employed as true intelligence and reason. We simply had not learned what to look for and how to interpret

the signs, since we hardly found references, or the right references, in the world around us. Now we begin to recognize, that we carry all of the references within us, so that by resonance with our surroundings, they may be aligned with real experiences. Hardly anyone has exemplified what true love really is. The subconscious has been trying all along to communicate, but we did not understand its language. Now we are remembering, step by step, who we truly are. Thus we are invited to create and allow a much larger frame of reference within us and around us.

Our computer technology is an analogy that can guide us along. Our use of the internet can show us, how we deal with our inner connections. Our current definition of success drives us to produce software and consumer goods that are not compatible, making us believe that less money will be made if we create compatibility. Fear puts profit before collective collaboration and higher goals, and recognizes neither benefit nor meaning beyond the goal of profits. This is how misuse and the loss of trust come into play. What we think of the internet and how we use it, reflects our attitude about our own inner networks. It reflects also the way we use it and the connection to ourselves and to all that exists. Figuratively speaking, this means the concept of separateness.

Future

Apple founder Steve Jobs said in his famous speech at Stanford University: *"Don't let the noise of others' opinions drown out your own inner voice...and most important, have the courage to follow your heart and intuition. They somehow already know what you truly want to become."* It is quite possible that here, too, a significantly larger frame of reference can be found beyond the idea of an occupational profile, to answer the 'question of who or what we really want to be – that is, to become and be, who we are from the time of our birth. This is something that virtually all of us have experienced: the noise of voices from our childhood has drowned out our inner voice. This inner voice is our intuition. Albert Einstein developed the basis of his theories not from scientific analysis only, but from intuition and gut feeling as well. There are countless quotes attributed to him that point the way to a completely different future in which we will not be happy as long as there is one unhappy child on this earth. Evidently this wise man understood something highly significant – that we are all connected. Director Steven Spielberg has also mentioned intuition as one of the most important factors in his success. It is the voice that connects us to all other whispering voices in this web of energy, many of which we exclude because they are "poor" - let alone the whispering voices of animals, plants, trees, stones and whatever.

Under the definition of success as we know it, our impression leads us to believe that little material wealth equals little wealth of the heart. Strangely enough, poor people are often much more willing to give what they have than those, who have a great deal. How else could it be that an average of 5% of people on this earth own 95% of the wealth, yet do little to change the conditions in this world? Therefore, the statement that little outer wealth points to unsuccessful people with little inner wealth is basically invalid, yet most of us still believe and justify our actions with exactly that statement. Could the reverse be true? Is this why we are so afraid of our whisper voice, because it would cause a change with all consequences, and might uncover our misunderstood beliefs about wealth?

Potential

Telepathy is the word of the hour, although it was considered to be smoke and mirrors for the longest time. Telepathy is nothing else but the subconscious mind being connected to the subconscious mind of someone else. Yet it is so much more, for it is not just our fellow man that has a subconscious mind. The subconscious and consciousness are just the energy of another, larger consciousness, and all of it represents the same energy in a myriad of ways. Everything on this planet is made of this energy. The entire universe is made of this energy, and if we want to believe what some have said, there are myriads of universes beyond ours, which are also made of this energy.

Through intuition, love forms a dedicated line to all information that has ever existed – everything that ever was, is or will ever be. Everything already exists now in the eternal moment of now. The more we embark on the path to ourselves, the more we will automatically be able to enjoy these abilities. It is proper handling that is sometimes challenging for each individual. We are on new territory; nevertheless, practice makes perfect. This new territory is so new only, because we have not learned to maneuver through it from the beginning. On the contrary: we were actually encouraged not to believe in it. How often do we assume that children have a runaway imagination? How many people have landed in institutions on account of mental disorders? How many were misunderstood for the gifts they had? And how many were burned at the stake for such abilities in times long past? These are not the best conditions for the further development of such abilities.

Divinipotence literally taken shows the way back to light. If we can accept our true divine origin, the true potentials will become visible and the light in everything that surrounds us can be seen and felt, as it is simply the reflection of what we have found and accepted within ourselves.
When clairvoyance and psychic sensitivity connect us with the energies that have always been and will always be a part of us, we are justified in the hope and assumption that, in order to experience duality, we no longer need to constantly re-create negative events. When access of information past the imagined limits is possible, we can allow ourselves to create paradise, although we are living in duality. From the point of view that

everything is correct and important, nightmares, violence in films, books, plays and games could have an entirely new meaning assigned to them. Maybe many dreams are not so much tools to process negative events, but are rather intended to let us FEEL the horrible things that might happen, or have happened, through past remembrance. Maybe films, books and other media were invented to make it much easier to experience negative things without having to reproduce them over and over in reality, as bitter experiences. This would mean, that other tools are also naturally available to us from a young age, rendering the need to create new evils in order to experience duality unnecessary. If we knew of these circumstances, we would then handle all these things quite differently, and prepare our children from an early age as to how to deal with and effectively use the media. If we use our abilities the way they were given to us at birth, we would be much more capable of comparing all previously created negative experiences without having to recreate them newly. We would be able to recognize, experience and understand ourselves as divine beings, without having to repeat the ineffable cycle of fear, pain and suffering.

Our brain and intellect becomes reason, when we live according to our divine origin and love. The brain thinks. The reason understands.
To engage our intellect or reason means, to allow self-awareness and to acknowledge our own divinity. This means acknowledging our connection to a divine energy as truth, which means the awareness, that we are connected to and responsible for everything. This Is Reason!
In my way of thinking this seems to be, what signifies the beginning of the use of our unused parts of the brain.
Then we understand ourselves as we are really meant to be. Then we understand others as they are really meant to be. Then we understand nature as it is really meant to be.
Then we understand the world as it is really meant to be. Then we understand the condition of this world and the resulting

message as it is really meant.
Then we understand the achievements as they are really meant to be.
Then we understand what to do to create heaven on earth, as it was always intended to be.
The purpose of the brain is to express intelligence and to be reason. Our destiny is to understand who we really are, and our calling is to live what we really are. Knowledge becomes certainty and the power of love. Each of us arrives at home within themselves. Together we arrive in paradise. We are home, at home in God.

WE ARE THE CHANGE THAT CHANGES THE WORLD!

6. Fantasy and Imagination

Fantasy, also called imagination, is the mind's "magic workshop" – a switchman for future success. In the magic workshop of imagination, literally everything is created that man is capable of. Everything we see today on this planet has been created by all of us collectively. What we have considered to be intellect, led us to our fantasies, plans and the results. Albert Einstein hit the nail on the head with very few words, when he coined the phrase, *"Imagination is more important than knowledge, for knowledge is limited..."* The uncertainty about our own self blocks us from the goal-oriented application of knowledge and imagination.

Earlier, our imaginative childish excesses and fantasies were curbed. Fantasy was by no means dispelled, but it was linked to negative images, fearful fantasies and a kind of knowledge, that is not based upon unconditional love. The inner longing for unlimited self-expression was linked to the limited knowledge that had always been the way it was - with growing disastrous consequences.

Prerequisites

Our imagination serves to give form or shape to our longing, which in turn can be put into action. This force emerges from us automatically, but mainly when the mind is heavily stimulated and a strong longing is produced. This great longing arises in widely varying ways. One well-known and common form of longing is the joy and enthusiasm over a thing. Love and the human union between man and woman can be the source of strong longing as well. Healthy and positive sexuality can be a true muse in the service of this creative power. Another form of access that is rapidly gaining popularity are seminars for personal development, where people come together that share the goal of creating positive change in their lives.

This creates a significantly higher level of energy and opens the door and facilitates access to the creative power of imagination.

The power of fear can also prompt us to become extremely creative and active; in this case it is the survival instinct, rooted in fear, that drives our energy toward imagination and action. Many examples of daily crisis situations, such as arguments, dramas, wars, torture methods, or mere films and books bear witness to this.

It is not true that we do not have imagination; it is just much more difficult to use it for positive results, when we are in a state of worry, grief, fear or stress. In these cases, we misuse this power to imagine the worst possible outcome of the situation we are facing. Thus it seems as though this potential is not accessible or is closed off, but it is really just being used incorrectly. If the original feeling of the fantasy is spurred by fear, even if this is subconscious or unrecognized, it will produce an unpleasant reality.

Hidden Truths

Despite our good intentions, our current view of success has led us to create the worldview as we know it today. As long as the blind spot for true self-awareness, true self-love and our divine universal origin still exists, this will be the logical consequence.

The opening to fear is like a black hole that threatens to devour and take over everything in its negativity, apparently leaving nothing behind. The opening to love also develops such a suction effect, and evidently the old can also not endure. Normally this creates fear again, and all too often people give preference to the safety of the familiar – even if it is less successful than we would like. An expansion of the perception of the divine universal origin can simultaneously bring awareness that something new, something different, something better will come, even if it is unclear what it may be. This expansion of perception is accompanied by an expansion of trust. This fullness is in turn perceived by the heart. It is somehow just a kind of deeply knowing „THAT" there is something new, a real solution, a path but not knowing „HOW", „WHEN", „WITH WHOM", „WHERE" and „WHY". The heart is and has always been connected to everything by intuition, what than can be perceived step by step, if we encourage us to follow our intuition. In progress of this process we are able to realize and find the answers for your „HOW", „WHEN", „WITH WHOM", „WHERE" and „WHY" just by entering the new way. It is like life proves itself, just by following and trusting the flow or stream of life itself. There are so many doorways to perceive and receive these messages and answers. Everything out there can give us answer, when we are quite aware in the moments of being, and take care for those moments, when something catches our attention. The heart is the navigator, and the imagination converts these impulses into pictures, which then become new truths and insights and therefore new goals emerge, from which new plans are made, which can then be turned into concrete new actions.

All of our lives we have trained this muscle, the power of imagination, without really being consciously aware of it. Just as in the world of sports, persistent training is what makes the performance. All of those years we have unconsciously trained our muscle of imagination, primarily for negative things, thus we perceive that while we attempt to create many good things, in the end it seems that the unpleasant things simply cannot be held at bay. It is the aim of this book to offer a new frame of reference for the muscle of imagination. From this new point of view, each can then decide whether it makes more sense for them or not. Our imagination muscle is powerful either way – we just have to decide HOW to use it and WHAT FOR.
To what end do we use our imagination and with it our energy – for fear or for love, for negative or positive purposes? For a

low-energy field or for a high-energy field? For blinders or for an expanded perception? For good health or for illness? For healthy relationships on all levels, or continued competition and battles? For a broken world or for paradise?

This era is one of the best ever for developing our power of imagination. At every corner we encounter new things, ideas and opportunities that stimulate our imagination. In the last 150 years alone, our imaginations have produced unbelievable growth. We have learned to control electromagnetic fields. We have discovered methods of communication that make it possible for us to communicate all around the globe without any significant time delays. If we are capable of such great achievements, it should almost be a piece of cake for us to attain control of our thoughts, feelings and actions, so that we can apply them in a truly positive manner. One would at least think so. But precisely those technological achievements are, what could be distracting us reflecting and researching who we really are and what we really want, because we live in a time of such rapid inner and outer change. Sometimes it seems as though there is simply no time to look inward for even one moment.

This seems to evoke a sense of fear or alarm in many people. Alarm, because we do not understand what those impending and necessary changes may involve and what consequences they will have. This state of not knowing is much like a big black hole, a gaping emptiness that may be very hard to bear and which naturally produces fear. So it seems much more pleasant to invest our imagination and fantasies in ever-newer updates for technology, toys, cars, decorative items, wellness, fashion and sundry folderol, along with their respective uses, rather than utilizing the power of imagination and our fantasies, individually and collectively, to create within us and around us that so-longed-for peace and the much-desired states of health, love and humanity. We don't seem to understand, that the longer this ignorance of our divine nature persists, the more and faster we will create the scenarios of doom from our movies, because we subconsciously do everything that makes these events inevitable and possible. We don't seem to have the slightest inkling of how powerful we really are.

Visions

"A substantially new manner of thinking is required if humankind is to survive." With these words, Einstein put our current challenges in a nutshell. What a new kind of thinking could create, is a shift of truth about what we call success and love, along with all the subsequent changes. If we understand with the heart and use our imagination and the corresponding feelings to know what a situation is supposed to look like, we can change it, and above all, take the necessary steps to implement that change. When we use our intellect coupled with unconditional love, we attain a completely new understanding of all that has surrounded us all of our lives. This new understanding is the foundation that can take our imagination so far to new heights.

At a global level we require something like the belief in and a vision of the best possible condition of our planet, humanity, the environment, and so on. If a concrete, positively felt image emerges, something to replace the negative image and fear, changes are possible in the areas of politics, religion and economics.

„The intellect has a sharp eye for methods and tools, but is blind to ends and values." –Albert Einstein

The main reason why our latest achievements and our current insights from religions seem to solve one of our challenges while creating ten more, is based on the misunderstandings of ourselves and success. Achievements and insights that do not spring from true love to ourselves and everything else, automatically lead to the point at which we recognize, what stands between us and our deep longing for peace and love. Regardless of what areas progress is made in, we need a WIN-WIN for our hearts and our minds; this will produce a WIN-WIN of values and goals with tools and methods.

Limitations and Possibilities

The only true limitation that exists lies in how we use our imagination, our fantasies, or our capacity for both. No new world can be created, if we cannot imagine any other definitions of ourselves and of success. If we take a trip to the world of sports, the importance of training our imagination becomes self-evident. Researchers have found, that athletes who perform imaginary training of their discipline – whether they are not playing due to an injury, or within the scope of mental preparation for a competition – they display nearly the same physical reaction as if they were physically engaged in the sport.

Accordingly, muscle loss as a result of sports injuries is significantly reduced through the use of imagination. This shows that we are always in good training in a figurative sense.

Metaphorically speaking humankind currently deal with something like an injury lay-off and it is time to do what fore we are here. It is up to us what fore we use this muscle. Will we use it furthermore for having in sight only the dilemma of our injury and stay „ill", with the consequence that life - and our planet - will go down the tubes, or will we use this muscle to build up a new way of life and face the challenges of life in an effective way?
Our imagination enables us to combine and organize known concepts, plans and ideas. New things can be created by combining experience, observation and collected knowledge in a

new way. It is precisely that ability that we need in order to create what we really want to see – in ourselves on an individual level and on our planet in the overall context. An expanded perception of imagination, combined with unconditional love, can help us make different decisions in conflict situations, because we evaluate the conflict in a completely different way. In this scenario there is no sense of guilt – there is, however, a responsibility that comes with this new perception. If our imagination reconnects with the very essence of the divine core, it will enable us to also connect with the divine infinite spirit, universe, or whatever we want to call this energy. That is the instance of intuition and inspiration, that enables us to recognize the deeper meaning in the things that surround us. It opens up new horizons in perception, so that we recognize our patterns in the surrounding world. This capability is also responsible for the fact, that we can find answers in things that have nothing to do with the original question. The objects or circumstances are removed from the respective context and evaluated on the basis of our own context. Truly new and fundamental ideas are received through this capacity or gift, just as it enables us to receive energy vibrations from other human beings or everything that exists.

Miracles become possible when we connect to others in this way and develop a common vision. To illustrate this power, I would like to share an impressive story from the book entitled "Think and Grow Rich" by Napoleon Hill.
This story is about a teacher and preacher named Dr. Gunsaulus. He had recognized early on, that the education system is not what it should be. He thought that he had some good ideas about how to improve on it, and wanted to establish a higher education system where he could apply his own concepts. However, this dream required a million dollars. He began to ponder how he could raise these funds. He pondered these thoughts for two years without finding a sensible solution for producing the million dollars. During this time, however, a burning desire

was created. One day he decided that he should no longer think about it, but take action. He decided to raise the money within one week's time. Clearly a completely crazy idea, but his burning desire and the decision to challenge the universe, so to speak, for a GOOD CAUSE, set something in motion to make the impossible happen. And so he began to act. He placed ads in newspapers, that he would hold a sermon under the title "If I Had a Million Dollars" this week. He then went to work on his sermon, which he found incredibly easy, since he had been mulling over the subject continuously for the past two years. On the day of the sermon he even forgot his prepared speech at home. So he stood in front of all those people and began to reveal his dream, speaking from his longing and his heart. He told them what he would do, if he had these million dollars. He described his plans. When the sermon was over, a man stood up and came up to Gunsaulus. This man was convinced that Gunsaulus could implement what he had been preaching, and gave him the million dollars the following day. This man was Phillipp D. Armour, and the Institution that was built was christened the Armour Institute of Technology. Gunsaulus had managed to achieve something that seemed impossible in a very short time. When the unshakable conviction and a concrete plan to implement it has been created, his goal was attained within 36 hours.

It would be disastrous to claim that the two years prior had been wasted. NO – those two years were precisely what was needed to allow the passion to grow. They were necessary to create a complete vision of what would be done with this money and to allow the thought energy to solidify more and more. These two years were important, so that he could deliver his sermon so passionately; that his plans had energy, and the potential for change became evident. He had spent hours upon hours making plans. He had a picture in his mind and in his heart. He had goals in mind. He knew what he wanted and what he wanted it for. Through his inner passion he was able to light the fire in other minds. In Mr. Armour, he found the man who not only had the inner passion and was convinced, but also had the financial means available. Many others in Gunsaulus's place would have given up. Instead, he was able to experience a universal truth, from which Goethe spoke in his poem, The Essence of Commitment:

"Until one is committed, there is hesitancy, the chance to draw back and always incapacitation. Concerning all acts of initiative and creation, there is one elementary truth. The ignorance of it kills countless ideas and splendid plans: and that is, that in the moment when someone is finally committed, it also keeps the Divine Providence feeder. All sorts of things occur to help that person, that would never otherwise have occurred. A whole stream of events issues from the decision, raising in one's favor all manner of unforeseen incidents and meetings and material assistance, which no man could have dreamed of would have come his way. Whatever you can do, or dream you can do, begin it. Boldness has genius, power, and magic in it. Begin it now."

The Essence of Responsibility

Everyone who wants to DO and CHANGE something successfully knows, that it is the idea behind the idea that matters. This is the idea that results in the ACTION and the CHANGE with joy and energy. Gunsaulus had recognized how he wanted to apply his knowledge and his energy for the good of others, and how he could do it. He did not fight a deficiency in the education system, but rather designed a vision and a plan that showed, what he would change.

First there is the opportunity to create change. But without the determination, the clarity of the intention, the desire to reach the goal and the persistent effort all the way to the goal, even the best idea and the best opportunity is worthless. A burning desire, a deep inner longing and a certainty, almost obsession sometimes, is necessary to keep us going during the difficult times. At first it may be that the idea has to be nurtured along, for the inner impressions are strong. By and by the idea begins to develop its own momentum, begins to grow and nurture ourselves, because positive interim results are pointing toward success. Nothing drives success as well as success itself. This story does not tell us what happened after that. But I am certain, that the path to final completion of the educational institution presented Gunsaulus several additional challenges.

Finally, the idea will drive the intention and nurture it along. That is the nature of ideas. First we give them life, direction, guidance and movement, and at some point they develop their own momentum, so that they give us life, direction, guidance, movement and certainty. To what extent do we have a burning desire to change our own live? To what extent is humanity ready to change the conditions in this world?

When we use all of our knowledge for our very own expression of our divinity, the certainty finally could arise what we long for: self-assurance. Out of the desired trust comes the trust in ourselves, and from the desired guidance finally divine (self-) guidance. Life can lead to fulfillment at last, because we are fulfilling life with who and what we truly are.

Ideas are energy and have much more power at their disposal than the one from which they came. They continue on long after their creator has died. In their smaller scale as convictions, beliefs and memories, and on a larger scale as religions, social structures, scientific achievements, artistic outpourings and much more. These ideas will continue to develop, on and on. Whether they serve the weal or woe of mankind depends upon the basic intention – fear or love. This also determines the nature of the respective changes and continued development.

Professor Hans-Jörg Bullinger, President of the Fraunhofer Society, wrote an article on the subject of imagination in the German daily newspaper, Süddeutsche Zeitung, on Friday, July 15,

2011, in which he stated that we have immense challenges to tackle by 2050. Bullinger explained that the annual need for raw materials will triple to 140 billion tons. The reasons for this are the growth in world population from the current figure of 7 to about 10 billion people, as well as the immense economic development in Asia and the African continent. The energy crisis and climate change are not the only problems we have to face – other answers must also be found. Our society is confronted with debt crises, over-aging, exploding healthcare costs, traffic problems, terrorist attacks, an increase in environmental catastrophes, etc. In their study, the Frauenhofer Society describes, that we need visions to tackle these problems.

Our society needs visions and people with unswerving belief in these visions who will turn them into reality, in order to not only manage or deal the problems but rather to solve these problems.

7. Action

Success as we know it is closely linked to ACTION. It is said, that the more you can do in a shorter period of time, the more results you will have. This is precisely what has caused the hamster wheel to spin faster and faster in recent years, while there seems to be hardly any time to pause and reflect. The consequences of stress have stretched us to or even over our limits, making ourselves smaller, lesser and weaker for this misguided process we call life, which seems to have little or nothing to do with who we really are. Our children, partners, families and friends experience these effects in our immediate environment while our colleagues, bosses and employees are effected in our wider environment. In the largest frame, these effects people at the very other end of our planet, which seems to have nothing to do with all our stuff, not to mention of our environment.

Peculiarities

As I write, I am surrounded by the spirit of Advent, a ritual brought to life by religion. Basically, this is a really beautiful and valuable time with an important message, prompting us to think about how we can express our love to whom. We wait for the light – simply beautiful.
We think about Christmas presents, decorations, whether we want to use the ornaments from last year or follow the new color trends; we ponder whom we want to invite or visit, what cookies we will bake and are annoyed, once again, that there are so many appointments during this time intended for reflection. Not a trace of contemplation, although the season evokes the desire to do so. In German „Besinnung" is contemplation and the part of that word „Sinn" means „sense" or „purpose" - but what is the purpose of all our humanity? Advent – a time of special lights, a time of charity and all of humanity. Economics and consumption seem to run rampant, drowning

out these high and mighty goals, and thousands of people will still starve to death during this time, while we ponder, what kind of cookies we will bake and what toys we might still be able to stuff into our children's overfilled rooms.

Please forgive this strongly polarized description about these observations, but that is precisely what is happening. The misinterpretation of success, which has apparently caused us to lose the real connection to our divine roots, actually leads us to believe, that this is all okay and that there is really nothing we can do about it. WE DO NOT CONTEMPLATE and step back to the real sense or purpose. Where is there true charity, real altruism and humanity? How long do we want to wait for Christmas, Christ's return, and the Divine? What are we waiting for? We are already there! What signals do we send to ourselves and our children? What are they learning from us about life, when we act this way and change nothing, even though we see it? What will they think of us one day, when they recognize and change what we did not want to change because our misunderstanding of success, power, wealth and separateness kept us from doing so?

Cause

Our daily actions and what we call successful is based upon plans dictated by politics, economics and religion. Especially the economy with its planning tools can give us some very useful hints. The necessary elements of a plan are: Goal, Review, Control, Correction and Execution.
This short list reveals the foundation of the rat race. We function in this process as an agency for the results. We are scheduled by the misunderstood successes in the areas of economics, politics and religion - that are likely to soon superseded by science and research as a new golden calf - something essential has been overlooked and short-changed. Since the point of organized ACTION is very important, I will address this in

more detail, beginning with the following (translated) quote:
„Compared to the ability to organize a single day's work reasonably, everything else in life is child's play." –J. W. von Goethe

The emphasis here is on REASONABLY. So far, the highest goal of success was the result, generally as a materially measurable unit intended to show "more of something", such as money, for example. All ideas, planning processes, procedures and results were aligned with this definition of the goal.
What would the "more" be, if we had a new definition of success and the entire process could be brought into alignment with our universal divine origin? Could it be that we would "produce" significantly more love, more positive energy, peace, affluence, health and growth? At this point we could justifiably ask the honest question: do we really want a peaceful, loving and healthy world? Do we really want it, or are we just lying to ourselves in order to ease our guilty conscience, so that we can further indulge in all of our material wealth? If we answer YES to these questions, Goethe's poem may point to something very important – the PURPOSE or MEANING.

As soon as we give this planning-process an entirely new meaning, other ideas, fantasies, plans and actions will appear. If we focus on the success of the soul's self-expression as unconditional loving, divine being and place all other goals in religion, politics, economics, science and research behind it, the entire sequential structure changes and reorients itself. The existing structures of our habits are not totally wrong, but rather require a review, control and in many cases a course-correction under the new awareness, with regard to newly prioritized values. That which has taken top priority up to now will not be completely discarded, but the priority of those values is corrected „downward". Therefore, the old behaviors will only be used differently but in a way that truly makes sense in terms of the newly appointed values. We could say that in this way something like "holistic" success might become possible.

A Different Way of Doing

Our entire life is ACTION, always... Even omission is an active form of NON-ACTION, and often non-actions are the most important action of all, at least in terms of the objectives of unconditional love, unconditional health and unconditional peace. They are namely the one, that has been so long overlooked and forgotten. We are always ACTING, no matter what. There is no such thing than non-action. It is only the question of whether what we think, speak, invent and do (= act) is either based on conditional or unconditional attitude and therefore objective - the differences in the results could not be more different.

If we consider the condition we ourselves are in, it seems eminently advisable to flirt more often with NON-ACTION, instead of jumping onto the daily hamster wheel. This would not only be beneficial for our own health; it would also allow us to become aware of the meaningfulness or lack thereof. It would also create time and space to become aware of our intuitive nature, which is all too often drowned out by the noise of our daily hustle and bustle.

There is much we should simply stop doing, if we really care about love, health and peace. That would give an entirely new value to NON-ACTION of conditional love, because this becomes so to speak the real ACTION of unconditional love.

The Why

As we heard above, NON-ACTION is basically something that doesn't really exist, since we are always doing something else instead.

Those who have more success according to our old interpretation of success just know what they want, have their visions, believe in them, and turn their goals and plans into action. They know exactly what they have to DO or NOT TO DO in order to reach their goal. As long as we do not actively plan FOR ourselves, we will be someone who is in the service of others, helping them to fulfill their desires, at the expense of our own desires and goals. Interestingly enough, it looks like about 5% of people are in control over that what seems to happen in this world. These are exactly the 5% who own 95% of the wealth on this earth. But what could be, if we create a goal that is bigger than our known goal of common success, which, however, this still involves?

What would be possible when we all would be able to recognize who we really are and how powerful we could be together, if the goals of these 5% and the action of those 95% would orient on unconditional love, health and peace?

Let us pose the question once more: Do we really want peace, health and love, for ourselves, our environment and the whole world?

The Consequence

Someone who is truly aware of themselves as divine being will be true to their desires, goals and visions and therefore their destiny, and have the need to be helpful to others to reach their goals and wishes. Like attracts like. Now, you may rightfully say, "But I don't even know my destiny!"

That's true, and not true. Until now! To be exact, many have a feeling of the way to their destiny, but the overall framework of our world could not show the background we would need to truly uncover the destiny, and therefore we began to doubt ourselves and so we did not make an effort to lend those visions, desires and goals as much expression as would be required to bring forth our destiny.

When we are true to our future self, we are also true to our destiny. Dreams, visions, desires and longings are the navigator. If we are true to our past self, something interesting happens, namely that which has always happened: we continue to think what we have always thought, continue to feel what we have always felt, say what we have always said AND do and don't do what we have always done or not done. We continue to have the same life we have always had, with the same „failures" we know very well. HOW IS THIS INTERESTING? NOW ... If we have NO interest in what has NOT worked all along, failing to satisfy our deepest longing for understanding, peace, love, good health and true communion and harmony, then we CANNOT find out WHAT works. The solution is already embedded in the challenge. We do not see it, because we have not made the effort to really look for it, and especially to accept the insights about what simply does NOT work.

Details

Let's look at the action and planning a little more closely. Individual steps of our plans become visible through our imagination. Plans are the tool with which we design HOW we are going to reach our goal. They also serve as guidelines, so that nothing is forgotten and, as an orientation for review, and thus quality control. It is indeed interesting that while we have mastered the basic process, we misunderstood its use.

Positive success depends to a great extent on HOW our daily ACTIONS are planned and how we implement these ACTIONS. By simply doing what has to be done and is required, we can attain superficial success according to the old definition, but we will rarely be truly satisfied with the results, let alone happy. Why? Well, no matter how you look at it, the life most of us live is not in harmony with our true BEING.

The 72-Hour Rule

Changes always begin with the first step, and therefore the 72-hour rule is important. It says that the first step should occur within 72 hours of the birth of an idea, if we want to have a chance of turning it into reality. Observations in the areas of personal development and success development have shown that things that are put into action within 72 hours have about a 99% chance of success. Conversely, we can conclude with a fair amount of certainty, that everything that is not begun within 72 hours has relatively little chance of success.

The first and most important step is to write down an impulse for change and write down goals and plans. We live in a world where bureaucracy seems to increasingly emulate madness, while the truly important things fall into the cracks. The reluctance to record our impulses, goals and plans is quite normal because we are overwhelmed with text and tasks.

Priorities

Priorities guide us through life and direct our actions. When we look at our daily life, we often realize, that what is important to us unfortunately does not have the priority we would like to give it. All too often, the structures of our close relationships deteriorate. because our success-oriented system dictates other structures. A change in our ACTIONS based on a new definition of success is surely the most courageous step mankind will ever take. All the more important, then, to be aware of the purpose.
An actionable plan design is required – one that includes how we will reach our desired goal, for the global situation has more to do with our personal dilemmas than we previously suspected. Our thought system should focus less on new plans that are intellectually-based, for these would be based on misconceptions and misunderstandings, since the intellect still operates in the old, deep-rooted misunderstanding and the resulting experiences of conditional success for reference. This prevents us today from using our erstwhile potential and genius. Rationality is trained to protect us from imagined emotional pain, that pain we experienced in our childhood through the withdrawal of love, when we did not follow the rules, denying us the experience of our own divine universal expression.

The Pareto Principle

The Pareto Principle states ,that 80% of success can be traced to 20% of the means applied. This means also, that 80% of the results are attained in 20% of the time. In order to attain 100% results, the remaining 80% of time would have to be used.

If we examine this principle, the question arises as to why in the world we do so much, running in circles of our daily rat race, and still not achieving what we set out to achieve. Moreover, it seems somehow logica, l that the way we think about success may have brought us to the point, where we are desperately trying to reach 100% - the misunderstood perfection - sacrificing our quality of life and our creative energy, all the while becoming less and less effective in terms of the actual goals of good health, peace, love and humanity. Is it possible that we are seeking perfection in the wrong place, when in fact it has always been present within us and in nature around us? Are we again trying to reach BEING through DOING, when it actually works the other way around? Could it be that precisely this is the reason that our days are so stressful and our life is the way it is, and our world looks the way it looks? If we can achieve 80% of what is important to us in 20% of our time, then why we don't do that? Again, a question arises: is what we're doing truly important?

Defeat as the Navigator

Defeat is an essential component of every plan and every life. It is a treasure trove that reveals knowledge and experience about expansion stages and upward capacities. Defeat will show us where the targeted goal is in harmony with ourselves and our overall objectives and where not.
Every change in values by which we assess our surroundings and ourselves, leads to a change in the habits.

So it is quite possible that a targeted goal, which was accurate prior to the inner change, suddenly is no longer in alignment with us ourselves, our overall objective, or even our planning. If we change our frame of reference for success and do or refrain from doing something out of unconditional love and self-realization, rather than out of the fear of loss, the priorities and expression of our goals may change dramatically. This can sometimes feel exhausting and can lead to self-doubt. Quite a few might then choose to acknowledge defeat – defeat through themselves, the circumstances, or other people and life in general, for such a drastic change in benchmarks may feel as though we are losing ground, will fall and maybe lose everything. But remember: first of all, it only feels that way and secondly, nobody is ever defeated until they give up.

Giving up happens in our head and for many it is even an affirmed thinking habit, as it reflects the inability to express oneself. Belief-based phrases such as "I can't do it", "that's impossible" or "this makes no sense at all" are relicts from times past and seem to substantiate our inability to change the condition of this world. All too often such messages appear just before we reach our goal. The process of change can be compared to giving birth. Some women experience heavy contractions up until just before the child is born, and this is the phase where they would rather just forget the whole thing, because they have the feeling, that they can't do it and it's no use. Someone else should finish the job.
But as we all know, bailing out during the birth process, or during one's own process of living, is not an option. Regarding our life, in the careful review of our goals, plans, their execution and the reasons for a defeat, we are confronted with an aspect of ourselves that is responsible for the failure – something we would like rather not see. This requires the willingness to look behind excuses, evasions and accusations. Anyone that devel-

ops this ability can discover behind the misinterpretation of failure the own potential, which can quickly reveal the sense of the current situation.

The Power of Change

"You must be the change you wish to see in the world." This phrase coined by Gandhi shows how important inner guidance really is. Change requires power and is created by the coordination of internal and external collaboration of our own parts, as well as the world around us.

A good leader is a person that can lead themselves. Our own personality aspects are guided so well that the true power of change becomes visible from within us – our own SELF. But how can we guide ourselves such, that the essential characteristics of our nature come to light?

There are two leadership styles: The Cooperative Style with leading by agreement and willingness to cooperate and the Authoritarian Style with leading by force.

Leadership by force and authoritarianism is no longer sustainable over time. Anyone wishing to ignore this has little chance of success, regardless of how big or how small their objective may be. A change in this regard is extremely important, especially for our own guidance. Since leadership through pressure is what we have learned and experienced so often through our environment, we end up using it automatically on ourselves. Ranting, punishing, sanctions and deprivation are expressions of this style of leadership.

Cooperative leadership is by far the most effective leadership style. Our world has entered an era where a new type of leadership style is required, even demanded, in all areas. The interesting thing about cooperative leadership is, that it displays many feminine qualities. While figures, data and facts are still important, emotions also play an important role. Particularly for sympathy and empathy, as well as the courage to take on responsibility and the capacity for teamwork, emotions seem to be increasingly important. Anyone that is not capable of channeling their emotions in appropriate and target-oriented actions rather than wielding authoritative power, will sooner or later have squandered their success. When someone can effectively manage their own and others' emotions, they keep sight of the big picture and – most importantly – their eye on the goal. This leadership style is directed at maintaining personal relationships and typically prefers a flat command structure. It displays more sensitivity and, above all, less control. At the same time the leader is aware of the importance of the little details that are often overlooked, and weal and woe of several goals are heavily dependent on noticing them. All employees are familiar with their common goal as a team. Everyone participates in reaching the goal, but the HOW is not so strictly predefined, allowing for more operative freedom as long as the desired result is achieved. Each participant's sense of self-worth, motivation and appreciation is clearly increased. There is a sense of a common mission to which each individual makes an important contribution. Thus each individual team member sees more purpose and meaning in the goal itself, as well as in their individual contribution. The quality of each participant's actions increases steadily. Setbacks are borne jointly. If this type of leadership style is consistently applied, it will generate more and more motivation, inspiration and courage to handle upcoming challenges. A sense of "united we are strong" and "together we can do it" arises. Trust and pride in action are the pioneer's or leader's boon if he chooses and upholds this leadership style. If we consider this with the goal of reaching paradise in mind, supported by a redefinition of success, we begin to sense that life could indeed be significantly easier.

Actionable Plans

Let's do a little experiment in thinking.
Let's assume that we place our divine loving self at the forefront for 365 days, and express ourselves in this way. We would allow ourselves to truly reflect and invest our time in profound honesty with ourselves, in order to make the changes that must occur.

What would be possible if we only use 20 % of all our daily means to create still 80 % of our daily success and use the other 80 % of our daily means for what is really necessary?

What would be possible, if we allow ourselves to give all the money that is spent on the production of decorative items, plus the money we spend as buyers, to those who have no food, clothing or roof over their heads – regardless of their location? What would be possible if we, who have so much already, would allow ourselves to donate the money to those who have nothing?

What would be possible, if we could allow ourselves to donate only half of all of the food in storage to those who are starving in the world? How much food would that be and how long would it last?

What would be possible, if we could allow ourselves to suspend all the large sporting events, along with all related measures, for just one year and use the money, time and resources saved, to take care of the real challenges we are facing in this world and in this era?

What would be possible, if we could allow ourselves to give the annual budget for weapons, military and defense of all countries lower priority and use 80% of the money to promote peace, health, altruism and charity, for just one year?

What would be possible, if we could allow ourselves to remove all foods, products and substances such as drugs, cigarettes, alcohol, and so forth that are not beneficial to our health in the causal sense, from the markets during that time? What would be possible, if we could allow ourselves at the same time to sell all organic and truly healthy foods and food products and other products at the same – or even lower – prices than conventional products?

What would be possible, if we could allow ourselves to share our abundance with all those people living on street, having no clothes, no home and no money, just by giving them what we think by our intuition would serve them in that moment we meet each other. What would be possible, if we could allow ourselves to suspend our luxury oriented thinking, with all of its consequences, for one year and allow ourselves the luxury of true humanity?

What would be possible if we could allow ourselves to live real equality regarding the tax laws? Everybody has to pay his taxes without using loopholes of tax legislation and tax havens. The amount of money hoarded each year at this tax havens could finance the survival of the 80 % of the people in our entire world, living with less than 10 $ a day also for 1 year, just by paying taxes like everybody else. What would be possible if only one year the money of the maximum earners, bunked in tax havens have to be payed like the taxes everybody has to pay. How much money would this be? How much would this relief the tax burden of the low and medial earner? How much national dept could be reduced this way?

What would be possible if a pay rise or a pension increase would not occur in percentage steps, benefitting those who already have more or even a lot, while those with less can't benefit of this regulation. What would be possible if everybody would get the same amount of money in such a case, no matter if you get a low or high salary or pension? How fast would the gap between rich and poor would be compensable?

What if we would allow ourselves to use the research funds for space missions, that are intended to make our continuation as a species possible, for research on how to preserve our own planet, and to first invest in other projects, when the challenges we are facing on this planet have been truly satisfactorily mastered? How much money would that be, and what would it make possible?

What would be possible, if we could allow ourselves to put to use all of the already existing wonderful achievements in the aspects of science and research, that were unwanted by the economy due to the fear of lost profits were dusted off? What would be possible, if we could allow ourselves to choose only those achievements as standard, which serve true health and the health of our environment?

What would be possible, if we could allow ourselves to make our health system not only affordable for those, who have enough money but also affordable for everyone? What would be possible, if we could allow ourselves to accept and promote or support the already quite good methods, which serves for unconditional health, which were not well received until now?

What would be possible, if we could allow ourselves to spend the whole generated amount of all our bonus and profit systems in total to give those who have very little or nothing to survive, rather give it back to those that revel in abundance anyway. We also could use this amount of money to face the worldwide ecological challenges.

These are only a few examples what human kind could change. What would be possible, if we could allow ourselves to realize that true health, true love and true peace is not about success and money but about the relationship of all of us as human beings and just one part of the expression of the holy divine energy?

What would be possible, if we could allow us, just for 365 days, to behave as people who have recognized that they are beings of divine universal origin?

How much time, manpower, reflection, aid, development, change and monetary potential would suddenly be made available, if we just once did not place success as we know it at the center of our existence? What could we change collectively, if we could allow us to use these freed-up resources uncompromisingly for the benefit of peace, health and humanity?

There are so many precedents on earth that show and bear witness that it can work in another way: whether pilot experiments in agribusiness or other educational systems - or even the dropouts, which demonstrates, that they nevertheless are able to make a good graduation or may even can make a meaningful contribution without going to school. There are cures that address at the root or there are people which are able to feed on light, etc. There are countless examples that show us, that there is another, easier and much bigger and better way.
What prevents us from accepting and using these innovations, after all they are serving our goals of health, peace and love? Why do we choose those innovations, which are causally an obstacle to these goals?

"To live is to change, and to be perfect is to have changed often." –John H. Newman (Cardinal, Roman Catholic Church)

The courage to fundamentally change can automatically bring about so many changes that it gives us what we no longer believed in: a "perfect" world of divine universal order. We already know that plants not have to go to school in order to become the best plant. No animal has to learn social behavior in its original environment, if it is allowed to develop naturally. No drop of water must be taught how to flow downhill or merge with a river, nor must it learn how to change its physical properties under the influence of the sun and heat. Cycles upon cycles that function perfectly. Why should it be any different with human beings? Could it be, that we all know at the bottom of our soul how life and success can work in harmony with everything, and that we are currently simply standing in our own way with our old misinterpretations and petty ways of thinking?

When we are truly self-aware, our entire being wants to express such a fundamental attitude day and night. Our actions will be one with our true self. Maybe we can now recognize, that the time has come to allow the most important ACTION of all to prevail: FORBEARANCE. It seems it is time to allow the flow of life, love, harmony, peace and health to happen naturally.

8. The Subconscious

All of the thoughts, experiences, and truths we have witnessed in life are stored in our subconscious, including those regarding success and failure. The subconscious is the connection and interface between all those things and our divine truth, because all experiences of our soul are also available through it, even if we hardly seem to have realized that until now.

Our subconscious is always active, it never "sleeps" or goes on vacation. Instead, it operates like a machine that is always ready and working. Unless we actively tend to positive in- and output, our machine keeps running automatically with the outdated data we have accumulated over decades, as well as information that is absorbed newly every day from our environment – the media, people, workplace, etc.

The output of our words and deeds lay in the quality of the thoughts and the corresponding feelings. The number of positive feelings that are present are directly correlated to the definition of success and our past experiences. What is in the foreground, however, automatically guides the purposefulness and focus of the subconscious. Nonetheless, both polarities - positive and negative - lack the fundamental connection between success and our divine universal origin and thus love. When scarcity is the main focus, the negative messages from our environment gain more access and weight than the positive ones. That dynamic is supported, for example, if one falls asleep or awakens to the TV or radio. The subconscious is wide open like a barn door, when we are in the state between waking consciousness and sleep. Any messages that enter unfiltered in this state play a powerful role in determining our internal orientation or amplifying any existing orientation.

Effects

The greater our desire to experience positive things is, the more we pay attention to positive in- and output. When this desire is lacking, the negative born of our misinterpretations will automatically occupy that space. If we take any random situation, a person who is positively oriented will look at the situation positively, while another person who is experiencing the exact same thing and has not established a desire for the positive will have a negative experience.

Everything that humanity has ever accomplished and will ever accomplish begins with a simple impulse of thought. At this point we allow ourselves to question, "How many people check their thoughts for validity, possibility and origin? Who has ever truly dared to fundamentally question the definition of success and life the way we are living it?"

It is our job to consciously and continuously check our negative thoughts and replace them with positive ones. The greater our desire for self-realization, self-love, self-consciousness and the self-expression that follows, the better this works. This ability is the key to the gate of the subconscious, because it allows us to see the purpose behind seemingly negative things. The subconscious creates our reality. That does not mean that it is reality itself, but rather that it represents reality, much like a sculpture or a painting depicts something. It creates an external image of what we think, believe and hold truth internally. The quote from American author, Anaïs Nin (which is often credited to Carl Gustav Jung), *"We do not see the world the way it is, we see it as we are."* fits very well here and should prompt us to ask ourselves exactly, how we see ourselves to have created a world filled with such separation, strife, destruction and apparent scarcity. As soon as we become clear about ourselves, we will realize the potential of change within us.

Abuse

Study and exploration in the field of brain research has made remarkable progress in recent years. This becomes evident in the way advertising materials are being used. We know how certain parts of our subconscious are wired, what stimuli we react to and which keywords it takes for a human being to react positively, e.g. "I want that". In the context of our misinterpretation of success, however, this knowledge is being abused in order to make profit.

Abuse in this context does not mean what the word typically implies, but points to the missing basis of divine unconditional love. If we put divine universal provenance as a value above the value of profit, we would have quite a useful tool to influence people positively in the sense of peace, love and order - divine order. A completely different profit could be realized here; profit that goes far beyond money and material goods, and which could not be bought with either.

The subconscious is the representation of and the interface to our divine origin, and to the misinterpretations, that where programmed by success and failure and which did and still do cause suffering. This is comparable to the picture of the golden Buddha entirely covered in a layer of mud. That mud represents all the pain and misinterpretations that have built up a protective armor around us. Without being aware of it, we have allowed our own definition of success to separate us from success and true happiness. Underneath we still are this whole, complete and divine being, carrying inside us all the knowledge of our divinity, including the knowledge of the divine universal order and the longing to live by it. Just as a drop of water contains the same structure and information as the ocean from which it originated, so does every human contain the knowledge and structure of the divine provenance and order within themselves.

Transformation

Once the crust of mud of misunderstandings is recognized, the divine starts shining through more and more. When we finally realize the greatest misunderstanding and allow change, that armor of mud can be cracked wide open quickly, for fundamentally everything we do is fueled by the longing for peace, health and love – our true origin.

Unique in all humans seems to be the need or desire to live by the divine order inherent in us all, which arises automatically once we begin to recognize and leave behind more and more of the old misinterpretations, misconceptions and pain. This need or desire arises, because we can then obviously recognize and express ourselves.
The need, to play the game by the rules, would be shared by everyone, because the ethics of our soul demands it. We are not referring to the rules, however, that have been written down in millionfold copy as laws, ordinances and commandments (most of these could indeed become obsolete); rather they are the rules of the divine order, that are found anchored deep within us and that render the behavior we observe today impossible, or only possible with massive emotional distress. Anyone who has attained a certain level of self-awareness cannot violate those universal rules any longer without being aware of causing themselves emotional pain. Essentially we could say that we simply have not yet understood what is causing this emotional pain that torments so many people.
So far it has not been possible to permanently establish this connection with the divine, since we have seen ourselves as separate from our divine origin, and were thus unable to make use of the information derived from our subconscious to recognize divine order as such and reestablish it within us. We have simply been oblivious to the rules, playing a game about which we had no clue. A change would now be possible, however, if we would only admit to ourselves, that we succumbed to a

massive fallacy – the fallacy of creating success on the basis of conditional love. We are capable of deliberately integrating any desired goal and any plan we wish to bring to fruition into our subconscious. It would therefore be desirable – and wise – to do so on the basis of our true origin. The following story illustrates the power of what we're referring to here:

"I walk down the street. There is a deep hole in the sidewalk. I fall in. I'm lost... I am hopeless. It is not my fault. It takes an endless time to find a way out.

I walk down the same street. There is a deep hole in the side walk. I pretend I don't see it. I fall in again. I can't believe I'm in the same place. But it isn't my fault. It still takes a long time to get out.

I walk down the same street. There is a deep hole in the sidewalk. I see it is there. I still fall in... it's a habit. My eyes are open. I know where I am. It is MY responsibility. I get out immediately. I'm walking down the same street. There's a deep hole in the sidewalk. I walk around it.

I walk down another street.

("Autobiography in Five Chapters" from Tibetan Book of Living and Dying by Sogyal Rinpoche, teacher of the Nyingma tradition in Tibetan Buddhism.)

The realization that we have simply misunderstood ourselves, success and everything connected with it for our entire lifetime could allow us to choose a different street, metaphorically speaking, and play the game of life with all its pertinent rules in a purposeful and goal-oriented fashion. One of the most important steps we must take to this end is, to trust that this new understanding of success can truly bring change. What good are words, tools and other forms of assistance, if we don't trust that they apply to us and will actually work? The interesting thing is, that anyone can try this out themselves to see that it works. Each new success in recognizing and remembering who we really are increases our confidence and a deep-seated knowledge of the rightness of our origin, thus increasing the odds for a positive and lasting change.

Nescience

"I want more success", "I'm for more peace", "More equality would be good", "I just want to be understood", "I just want to be happy".

We find such statements in different forms in all sorts of discussions among couples, parents and children, companies, unions, in politics, religion and economy. Where is the primary emotional focus in these statements? On the surface these statements look quite positive. But when we look closer we can detect something else. The driving force behind these statements is based in scarcity: not enough success, not enough peace, not enough equality, not enough understanding, not enough happiness. The responsibility is passed off to someone or something external. A clear message about what the goal is and what is necessary to reach it, is missing entirely. Therefore, the environment is forced to reflect those circumstances that represent, for example, scarcity of peace or too little equality, not being understood or unhappiness. We must begin to differentiate and think in an intentional manner for we are unwittingly co-creating these scarcity scenarios. Our environment can only support us in the fulfillment of our needs, when we know ourselves better. What we experience as negative in those situations is the attempt of our environment to reply unconsciously to unconscious messages. As long as we don't know who we truly are and what we truly want, our environment will be hard pressed to support us the way we want. We end up going in circles.

The subconscious and emotions

Emotions are like the breath of God that breathes life into everything we do. A few important positive emotions are:

love, gratitude, trust, desire, enthusiasm, hope, tenderness, etc. The more we incorporate those emotions into our lives, the more they act as magnets, attracting more positive emotions. The most important negative emotions are fear, hate, anger, jealousy, envy, etc. Fear is the antagonist of love but it also stems from love. Fear arises from the misunderstanding of conditional love compared to divine unconditional love, that was not reciprocated during childhood and subsequently misinterpreted. Fear demonstrates to us very clearly the misunderstanding of our divine primordial truth, that has come between our true expression and the expression we are "forced" to live. Hate is the strongest manifestation of fear and an expression of love being entirely incapable to find the target of its wishes or desire. In this case, self-expression does not produce the desired goal to be seen, accepted, recognized and loved.

It may be impossible for positive and negative feelings to fill our mind in equal amounts, but it is possible for negative and positive thoughts to exist at the same time. One of the two emotions takes over the lead, and it is our choice and responsibility which one we will express. We can choose to recognize our divinity and our oneness with all, or our separation from „God" and from all. We can choose success and the resulting actions based on understanding or on misunderstanding. We can choose success as a result or a reason. The end results could not be more different.

Access the universal source of knowledge

This part is basically so simple and yet so challenging: we can finally just listen! This statement is pointed out often in the books of Neale Donald Walsch „Conversation with God" as well as the statement, that we just got all wrong. This source has been talking to us the entire time – we just forgot how to listen. If we follow our inner voice instead of the old voices of our childhood that reverberate in everything that surrounds us, we can actually attain more and more self-awareness. It is time to pay close attention to that voice.

Intuition – the sixth sense

Everybody is familiar with sudden intuitions, epiphanies and déjà vus. A sudden knowledge of something we didn't think we knew appears, but until now we didn't know what to make of it other than that it sometimes saved us from harm or that we knew ahead of time who was calling before picking up.

In a commencement address at Stanford University, Steve Jobs expressed it this way: *"You can't connect the dots looking forward, you can only connect them looking backwards. So you have to trust that the dots will somehow connect in your future. You have to trust in something: your gut, destiny, life, karma, whatever. Because believing that the dots will connect down the road will give you the confidence to follow your heart, even when it leads you off the well-worn path."* However, this seems to be just the tip of the iceberg.

If we ask life concrete questions we get answers – inevitably – because everything is success, so life can but answer. The question is, however, do we recognize and understand the answers? To receive those answers, we need the sixth sense and the capacity for creative imagination and vision, for these answers appear "hidden" since we never learned how to use this sense of ours. The answers come in the form of feelings, inner pictures or movies, appearing in front of our inner eye, when our subconscious get in touch with something of our environment that contains our answer we are longing for. Intuition – that moment of recollection or primal memory of a connection between our own origin and our own purpose of existence – communicates through the feeling of immediate reconnection to the ubiquitous energy grid, which we experience as love, oneness, trust, knowledge and understanding. Here reveals the massive effect of the misunderstanding of „ALL IS ONE". If everything really is one, then, we after all should assume, that answers are not only found in books, films, science and research, but also in everything that surrounds us. Then it seems quite understandable that everything that ever was, is and will be, is to be found in any manner out there and in such a way that we can understand it. And here then closes the circle to „*The question is not who am I talking to, but who's listening*". As long as we do not believe that we are one through this divine universal primordial energy with everything that exists, we will not be able to enjoy to hear the answers of "God", much less we will understand our own life or life itself on this planet. And this leads us to: „*You got me all wrong*".

But this could change if we really start to believe what Shakespeare once already expressed: *"There are namely a lot more things in heaven and earth than we could imagine."*

Our ability to use our intuition or sixth sense grows automatically the more we are able to leave behind us the misinterpretations, false definitions and the perceived pain connected with them. This is accompanied by a different, "higher" form of energy, that allows us to translate the information from the normal external context of our environment and its challenges into the internal context of our soul and experience. We gain a bird's eye view of completely new and higher possibilities of perception, with which completely different correlations and thus pathways and solutions become visible and possible.

The expression of the sixth sense, or of that link with the universe and the divine or boundless mind, manifests in very multifaceted ways. This ability connects us with the web of energy surrounding everything and of which everything and everybody is a part of.

How the sixth sense is influenced

Intuition is significantly influenced by what we call our conscience. Our conscience as we know it, is fed on one hand by the connection to our divine core and on the other hand by the misinterpretations of our upbringing. The discrepancy between our divine core and those misinterpretations are experienced as a guilty conscience – the experienced conditional love and the unconditional love that our being is based upon are not congruent.

People who have brought about change all possess one important ability: they listen to intuition and trust the resulting ideas, which they then make real through relentless action on the outside, regardless of how many setbacks they experience, or other people that think they're insane. Genius comes more and more to light, the more we let go of past – often negative – experiences. Ideas born of creative imagination are much more reliable, since they come from the one great source – the divine core that lives in everything.

Genius

According to Wikipedia a genius is *"a person with outstanding creative mind power ("a brilliant scientist," "a brilliant artist") or even particularly outstanding achievements."* Originating in French and Latin roots it was once *"Generating force"* and in Greek it meant *„become, emerge"* then *"personal protective God"*, later *„anlage, talent")*

In this definition we recognize again the creative or primordial force that could be an inherent part of our success, if we defined it differently. It talks about BECOMING and EMERGING BEING and CREATE, even of a „personal protective God". Only later in the course of history this definition was reduced to less than it actually is. The terms "talent" and "anlage" implies, that genius is only accessible to a few select people, and assumes certain specific achievements. Reorienting what we call success would automatically connect us to that original interpretation of genius and have us become aware, that we all bear within us the talent of the divine and the unlimited and thus the genius.

This gift lies in every one of us – EVERYONE! We need to deploy our primordial force, because now more than ever, it takes a genius to master our daily conflicts and challenges in different ways than we did in the past, with completely new creativity and positive emotions. If we have the courage and the will to look at and acknowledge the fears hidden behind the false definition of success, our intuition can then guide us to the truth inside of us through our genius. This could result in us drawing our very own conclusions and discovering new solutions for ourselves and the challenges of our times.

The more often we use this ability, the more it establishes itself and becomes a habit or a natural part of us. All of our daily sorrows and problems are then still part of our lives, but they no longer cloud our view with fear and therefore no longer occur as an existential threat. The true divine connection can then actively work so that challenges appear in a different context and approach them differently.

The intellect is the tool capable of combining familiar experiences and knowledge newly and holistically to create a completely new possibility for solution, provided it is enriched with the knowledge and experience of the primordial being, unconditional love and the resulting approach to success. This could in fact be the solution to all of the great challenges of today's world.

The more people become aware of their inner genius, their true selves and, with that, their purpose here on earth, the more effectively the challenges of our current world can be solved. And they could be solved in a way that we cannot yet see, let alone surmise. These solutions lay beyond our current experiences and the related solution approaches can be found in our present underutilized areas of our brain.

Active use of a stroke of genius

A genius focuses on the known aspects associated with a challenge. A virtual picture is created which takes hold in the subconscious. This picture is underlined with the clear question, "How can this work?" This is where the Reticular Activating System comes into play. The RAS works like an antenna; it senses stimuli and alarms the brain to pay attention. In a sense, it receives a "search for solution" command and acts like a radar that now scans the personal reality for answers and puzzle pieces to the challenge.

With this process it is important to detach and release the mind from its focus on past definitions – in our case the definition of success and how we are used to experience our world. We can allow ourselves to detach and set ourselves free to think, perceive and do something completely different. Herein lay our chance to rethink and for change.

When we are ready to accept a new basic assumption, we simply have to "wait" for answers to spring into our mind. The answers themselves were already there; we simply could not see them, because the expansion of our horizon had not yet taken place. With that expansion of the horizon, our brain scans in new and different ways and consequently finds new and different points of view and possibilities for solutions. It can happen, when we're in the middle of a completely mundane task, that we suddenly discover, beyond that action, the solution hidden within it. The Noble laureate for chemistry, Kary Mullis, for example, discovered the principle of polymerase chain reaction (PCR) not in a laboratory but while driving on a freeway in Northern California. The results can occur instantly or delayed but they do increase the more we slow down our daily routine and go through it more consciously and aware. It is often thoughts that in a normal context are regarded as out of place or crazy, not unlike the ideas of well-known geniuses that in the beginning were often ridiculed or at times even opposed. Now that we have some knowledge about geniuses, we can possibly skip that part and proceed directly to supporting any person that has discovered their genius and manifests it on the outside with the welfare of all in mind.

Meditation

Meditation is a very powerful tool for a dialogue or a meeting with the great all-encompassing divine/mind/universe within us. The conscious mind communicates with the subconscious and thus also with the superconscious. Prayer basically serves the same purpose, although its use is often a bit misguided. We were taught to use this tool as the last straw and only when all else has failed, or we were taught to repeat a completely emotionless prefabricated prayer, that is completely disconnected from the purpose of life, rendering the act of praying virtually ineffective. If we pray out of pure fear and despair, it will rarely provide a positive answer, unless we detach from the fear, stand completely in our trust and can already feel the desired result. This is what is meant by the phrase, *"Your faith has healed you"*. Most of the time, though, the fear of loss clings to a particular, fixed and hoped-for result or, conversely, the absolutely worst possible outcome for the situation. Emotionless conversing on the other hand, as found in the prefabricated liturgical prayers and litanies, are but hollow noise. It has no soul.

If we use this instrument regularly it is a valuable aid in providing positive guidance. This allows us to receive answers through our feelings that we cannot hear with our normal ears and rarely see with our eyes. When the heart unites with the eyes and ears, we begin to recognize things beyond the context we have defined and are familiar with.
When we open up to this force and ourselves, we will suddenly see the answer we have so desperately been waiting for from our environment, for example from the fragment of a sentence

spoken by another person, that has nothing to do with us. It is equally possible that we hear the right song at the right time or read the right book, or even just one crucial sentence. Even the play of our children, looking at a sign or finding a rock can provide an answer if we see it with different eyes. The more we sensitize ourselves to the fact that an answer is far more than what we previously knew about prayer and meditation, the more likely we are to be able to detect it.

We can understand the answers – quite automatically. It is our natural born right to perceive things in this manner – life itself becomes more and more like a meditation; for meditation is not something we do but a state of being with heightened divine presence and perception. In the beginning this communication primarily demands trust, patience, perseverance, desire and the aforementioned understanding of our true origin.

The inner guidance or intuition is the connection to everything that exists, and it serves as a compass that leads us to the miracles of life. This energy lies far beyond what religion considers divine energy. The divine is everywhere and always.

Fear does not allow us to „listen", while love and trust do. The extent of our trust shows how much we already remember our true selves. Trust is the fundamental prerequisite for reconnecting, and the possibility that each one of us can contribute our genius, so that this world can be the paradise it actually always was.

"Find yourself, be true to yourself, learn to understand yourself, follow YOUR voice, only this way can you reach the pinnacle!"
Bettina v. Arnim, German author and key figure of the German Romanticism era

9. Self-Awareness

Self-awareness or self-knowledge are an indispensable ingredient of success because it results in the next better version of our self, along with the results produced by that new version. This new version of ourselves is significantly influenced by the way we view success. Self-awareness is the first step toward change. To produce change, we need four crucial elements: courage, trust, openness and honesty.

Self-awareness requires trusting ourselves and others in order to reveal ourselves the way we truly are, so that we can become the next improved version of ourselves. The progress of our self-awareness depends on the amount of trust we have in ourselves and how conscious we are of ourselves. Self-awareness and self-confidence are almost identical in their meaning, yet seem to be considered as completely different things in our speaking. In exchange we attempt to push self-love into the foreground. Self-love is actuality self-confidence, since that automatically accompanies love and therefore also self-love. Self-awareness rather seems to mean to recognize and accept our divine being wholeheartedly. Self-confidence is more likely to show how we live according to that and if we do so.

Self-Confidence

According to Wikipedia self-confidence is generally defined as *"being convinced of one's abilities, of one's value as a person, expressed typically through self-assured behavior. Colloquially, however, self-confidence is generally seen as a person's or group's feeling of positive value inside a context of social value. It is therefore often used as a synonym for the term self-esteem. High self-esteem is thus seen as high self-confidence or arrogance.*

Self-confidence always refers to a set of values and an environment that is giving approval or disapproval: in the first case self-confidence is determined by characteristics and abilities that more or less correspond to commonly held values; one is self-confident, if they feel acknowledged in regard to those values. **In this context, self-confidence usually refers to a precritical feeling of social self-value, that one either possesses or lacks, and which can be increased through acquiring socially desirable attributes (like collective consciousness, self-determination or personal responsibility), or diminished in case of failure.** *On the other hand, a person is also considered particularly self-confident, if they as an individual confront a group of people that conforms to certain values.*

This definition demonstrates the discrepancy between self-confidence, as well as self-awareness, and the true divine origin.

The Deeper Meaning

Self-confidence as we know it, e.g. as described in the first part of the definition above, is based on our misinterpretation of success. Self-confidence has been misinterpreted, since our previous definition merely entails to know one's strengths and weaknesses and to act positive-result-oriented whenever possible. In the original meaning of the German wording, however, self-confidence is the state of being aware of our true origin of divine and universal provenance and expressing that in our actions. With this awareness it becomes clear, that behind perceived weaknesses there are laying unrecognized potentials, revealing themselves more and more through our awareness alone.

In the sentence in bold type above we can detect the approach to our new definition of success, which is accompanied by an entirely new collective consciousness, real self-determination and true personal responsibility. When people are truly aware of their self and thus connected to their divine or universal core, they can't behave in another way than a social way. This social behavior goes far beyond what we currently live on this planet, because we still very much differentiate who is actually worthy of our sociality and, if so, of how much of it. This new social behavior is so deeply rooted in our inner self, that it would occur as self-harm to act against the environment, against other people, against animals, against economic principles and against ourselves out of the desire for material success.

There glimmers an authority within each one of us that demands this: the ethics of our soul. This authority is our measuring instrument, which evaluates whether something is in alignment with the divine universal order or not, and reveals the assessment to us through our feelings. We simply have not yet understood it.

Consequences

When we human beings would be truly and fully aware of our divine universal origin, we could indeed become present to our own power and – more importantly in our times – to our own responsibility. A compulsion in us could arise to change the world, because we feel the emotional pain caused by the condition we and this world are in.

Many seems to get stuck in the early stage of their development and on their way to self-awareness, because we just don't understand, what is causing us so much pain. An increasing number of us suffer from depression or choose suicide, or work ourselves to the point of burning out.

An expanded definition of success would result in us having an entirely different awareness of ourselves, our emotional pain, our depressions and the fears accompanying a burnout, which in turn would have as consequence, that the contact with the universal order through our innermost core alone would automatically empower us to be willing and able to our shortcomings.

With real consciousness and self-awareness of our true origin and potentials, we would neither need this ever-growing mass of laws nor the military and police. We would no longer need to protest for the environment or worry about our food being increasingly unhealthy.

Harmony with all that exists seems to be a deep-seated need of an awakened soul that is truly and fully aware of itself and, in the totality, the need of a collective of such souls. Such persons want to express through their own being who they truly are and they would suffer, if they act against their own inner divine universal nature. Self-aware people do whatever is needed, wherever it is needed, and when it is needed, to transform this world into that which it always has been – a paradise.

It is now up to us to decide, if we as humanity want to keep chiseling away at our true nature, suffering all this pain and misery, that we evoke and cause ourselves each and every day, or if we are ready to recognize ourselves as universal beings that are connected to everything, so that we may assume our responsibility and bring forth real change.

This transformation necessitates neither war nor more money. We simply have to bring forth the willingness to question what we have always believed to be true but which was built upon the misunderstanding of love and success. When we would be able to redefine success in a universal context, we would empower ourselves, individually and collectively, to change this world in a minimum of time. We already have all the means necessary to do this.

Evaluate Constantly, Never Condemn

Self-awareness and self-analysis is like meticulous detective work in which we discover our whole truth. It is quite possible that we stumble upon parts whose superficial truths we find embarrassing. Other parts will have us standing in front of ourselves muttering the words, "Oh my god, how could we think, talk and act that way without realizing it?" It doesn't matter – just keep looking. We actually empower ourselves when we recognize and acknowledge these uncomfortable parts as our own. We recognize the misinterpretation of our old thinking and can finally bring home the forgotten potential hiding behind it.

We are judge and jury. We twist and turn so as to see ourselves from all sides – as plaintiff, as defendant, as attorney and as defense counsel – but always without SELF-CONDEMNATION. This is not about judgment, but about the EVALUATION of whether our thinking, feeling, acting and speaking are consistent with our true divine universal BEING. We learn to evaluate, if that, which is going on within us, is beneficial to us and to those around us.
It is also not about giving up JUDGING entirely, but rather about turning judgment into an evaluation. To judge means to distance or separate ourselves from the primal part of the divine universal core that is omnipresent. Evaluating on the other hand recognizes that primal part in everything that is and remains or newly enters into contact with it. We then separate us from these behaviors, which are not in alignment with our divine universal core.

Evaluation is a process that permits us to allow and examine different points of view on neutral ground, and which makes our own new update possible through the inner resonance of intuition. The various opinions enable an ever-deeper understanding of being human and the patterns of thought, feeling, speech and action. They open up the depths of our perception of the connection between and among all things, thus opening the door to the divine universal truth.

This understanding could be the missing basis for change. It allows us to recognize the fear in ourselves and others, that prevents us from making a better decision for our benefit and for the benefit of our entire environment. Those who have increasingly resolved their fears will have a much easier time, recognizing these fears in others and encountering them with kindness and compassion, and we would become able to re-act in another way and therefore we could create another reality or outcome. We then become an example and let the divine energy, our light, shine from within us. The deeper we dive into our own SELF-UNDERSTANDING, the more we draw from the abundance and wealth present within us. Our fears block us from receiving that abundance and wealth, just as they do with the people around us.

The Law of Economics

This is the one instance that nobody escapes. This instance equalizes like an invisible eye or a jury. Everyone that does something meaningful is rewarded. Life is merciless, however, if we want to have abundance and love without giving abundance and love. It really is about time that we put the true meaning of life before material success, so that we can express as one who we really are, and experience harmony and inner wealth in conjunction with external wealth. Success as we have lived it until now is not wrong; it seems to be merely a small part of the whole truth about our original existence and, with that, about our real potential. There is simply something missing. Once we would be able to update our thinking about success, we would be able to indeed create a paradise. That would be true self-awareness and the biggest gift we could possibly give to ourselves.

10. Determination

Without determination, no success is possible, regardless of with or without a new definition and interpretation of success. We use this characteristic a thousand times each day for all those things that we subconsciously or consciously hold as true. We automatically make our everyday decisions on this basis. And one part of us upholds the old unquestioned standards and goals of our society with great determination. We forgot, that we once subconsciously set goals, based on the ignorance of our entire environment, regarding our true origin. The fear of loss of love, recognition, community, physical integrity, etc. is, what led to those goals that no longer serve us yet maintain their influence over our daily decisions. It's time to change, isn't it?

Effects

With great determination, paths are followed today that turn massive profit into even more profit. With equally great determination, the devastating effects on the environment and people, are being ignored. And with frightening determination, individuals are applying every bit of strength they can muster to get a piece of the pie, while free time, health and family life often are left behind.

With great determination we work to give our children a life that leaves them increasingly discontent, irritable and more difficult to influence. A life that already does not serve us. With well-meaning determination millions of dollars are senselessly spent from various annual budgets at the end of each year, because otherwise the budget will be lowered in the following year. With questionable determination vast amounts of food are destroyed every day, while in other places people dig leftovers out of the trash or even starve to death, just because our laws, rules and regulations state, that it is inhumane to use expired food, or that it is too costly to ship the food where it is needed, or that it would never get to where it is needed. And most of all for the reason of better prices. Where there is no will, there also is no way. What we are looking at here, is destruction of resources par excellence. In all of these seemingly unrelated results of what we call success we can recognize, that our thinking continuously shuts down the humanity, that is inherent in our divine universal nature. Words and letters on pieces of paper are more powerful than we human beings ourselves, writing them down there, prohibiting the needed humanity.

Our unconscious goals based on scarcity will remain in existence until we look at how we behave and why. Today we can choose newly. Our daily thoughts, actions and words show us what separates us from love, peace and fulfillment. We live our NOW unaware and judge many things from the perspective of the past of our human lives and history. Our NOW appear to be a reflection of what was in past. And exactly herein lay our chance. If we make our assessments from a conscious perspective of our eternal divine universal „past", our NOW can equally represent a mirror of what was expected, so that it would be paradise rather than hell on earth. We should merely use the „better" past, that really serves us.

Determination is the master of our procrastination. If we manage to put a leash on the latter, we have accomplished an important step on our path to success.

Determination has the characteristic that we decide very quickly and emphatically when we have a clear goal. Clear decisions in turn are the basic requirement for more success in life. So far profit has stood in the center as a clear goal, and this lead us to create a world that creates further progress with great determination, while our social and economic situations regress, as if two exclusivities are necessitating each another. This progress is important and right, and if we choose to, we can now realize that it does not have to continue at the expense of social, spiritual and environmental parameters.

On the contrary, it can bring holistic profit as long as we keep those parameters in the foreground. When we designate the new definition of success as a clear goal and put love, abundance, trust, peace and the best possible result for all at the center of success, we can use that same determination to create a completely new path with new priority goals, in which profit would acquire a new meaning but definitely not be short-changed. It is just very likely that we equally see profit in things outside of material wealth, obtain it and most importantly also enjoy it.

A Clear Decision

Clear decisions are characterized by the fact, that they only can be changed or adjusted very slowly. This is easily recognizable in the current debates about environmental protection, human rights or the struggle for economic growth at the expense of various factors. Our longstanding misinterpretation of success makes it extremely difficult to allow change, because the scope of perception, that would make it easier, was until now unavailable. The clear goal of safety and survival through the "success of the fittest" is so deeply anchored, that we haven't even been able to consider, that there may be a way which not only ensure survival, but also make it possible to live life in abundance.

A review of current goals, a setting of new goals and planning and execution of the plan are all-important elements for greater clarity. We have used these tools particularly in the great general context of economy and politics but without achieving truly satisfying results. Instead it seems as if humanity continues incessantly to turn in circles with its challenges. We would achieve dramatically different results, using these tools and steps, if we could change the basic definition of success. This newly obtained clarity could allow us to act with more determination in every aspect. This process is every bit as valid for every individual in the mastering of their own daily challenges, as it is for the large-scale challenges, this world faces each day. For the individual can only find their inner peace to a limited extent, if there is no real equivalent to be found in their external environment. We all feel increasingly that something is not right. More and more people are awakening, sensing their true roots and wishing to live accordingly.

With every new reiteration of this process, old misinterpretations are dispelled. As a result, the suffering resulting from the misinterpretations is healed. External circumstances want to show us, what is happening inside of us and how we are treating ourselves. They show us what can and should be changed.
When doubts arise, determination is indispensable. It takes great determination in challenging situations or when we have to fight old habits. It takes even more determination the more often we cross our own boundaries. When this happens, we feel the energy potential of the old habits adding up, so that it becomes increasingly difficult to live new habits – unless we discover the smallest common denominator. It takes a great deal of decisiveness to act differently in the moment of detecting the proverbial one-way street or the hole into which we could fall. When we notice that wall towards which we are walking, it takes all of our decision-making power to pause and stop ourselves. Today this figurative wall and this figurative hole are present to a high degree, and we notice how difficult it is for us to embark on new, different paths. We experience that every day anew with ourselves, with our environment and with the big picture.

Decision Guidance

When we encounter a lot of failure in our life, it is important to decide which voices we will trust and which we won't. When is it advisable to listen to others and when not? When is it more advisable to listen to ourselves and when not?
We have often had to learn, that things are worse than they

seem. This stems from having been punished and limited very often as children, although we just wanted to live out our own expression of life. This was the normal and logical consequence of taking the widely accepted definition of success for unquestionable truth. This definition makes us seem smaller and lesser than we are and things seem worse than they are. Unrealized potentials were and are on the daily agenda, because they don't fit the framework given by our worldview.

Interestingly, more and more of these unrealized abilities are documented in studies of quantum physics and brain research – thank God. The amount of people having "supernatural" experiences are on the rise. In the past, these people would have been burned at the stake. Today it merely makes life with others more difficult, since other people cannot and do not want to believe it, if they have not experienced these expanded perceptions and abilities themselves. Often they proceed with great determination against the new and for the old interpretation and definition of what we know. In this case it is advisable to listen to one's own voice. But it is also possible that we see ourselves as small, and enter an environment that ascribes to us a quality we previously never noticed in ourselves, or never believed in, because our old environment either didn't reflect it or even excluded us because of it. In that case it is indeed advisable to listen to the voices of the others – this new environment perceives something we cannot see or we take for granted, or even considered negative.

Criticism also wants to show us something that we can't or don't want to see. This is often unrecognizable, however, because of the manner in which we practice criticism. The outside environment uses criticism to point out an external or internal deficit. It is indeed possible that without knowing it, our HOW is really not OK, in spite of a basically good intention. Therefore, the situation is pointing out inner deficits, that are manifesting in the form of missing updates to our own divine inner truth.

Thus the criticism is a reflection of how we treat ourselves. It is important to examine our inner truth, as well as the external circumstances, and change them with determination.

Know What You Want

In order to make the right decision it is important to know what we really want and how we intend to obtain it. By knowing what we truly want we exclude certain patterns of thought, speech and behavior, resulting in our steps toward change. Children make excellent examples for determination. A child that desperately wants something, will pretty much utilize any means available. The child is determined to reach its goal and has a clear objective, as well as a whole range of measures it takes. Those measures often increase in intensity during their course, or the child already knows exactly which measure will work best. Depending on how often it has dealt with a situation and gathered experience from it, the child subconsciously follows this exact cycle: experience – review – reflection – new goals – action – experience – etc. As long as we are unaware of our divine core and thus of holistic success, we act like our children, who merely display our ways of acting in a much more unfiltered way. We will also pretty much use any means to experience what we previously considered to be successful, without ever really taking the negative consequences into account.

Important requirements for determination are active listening, heightened awareness, an overview of the things happening around us, remaining silent and speaking at the right time, gathering and evaluating information, and determined action best suited for our goals. Hardly anyone of us has experienced and learned this on our own, because our perception of success lead us running onto the rat race that seems to be in opposition to these things. Let us examine these five points.
Active listening requires the ability to be fully present with the person talking, without allowing our own experiences and

thoughts to run away with us. For this we require time, which seems to become increasingly scarce given all that is happening around us.

Although heightened awareness is possible nowadays for an increasing number of people, we are still like a developing country in this respect. The overview of our environment is made much more difficult because it is not really clear to what extent the media reports what is actually happening and how much it is manipulated in favor of the global political orientation toward success. It is much the same with marketing strategies in the economy; it seems that often only a part of the truth is being presented, allowing the threads of success and profit to be further more intensively and invisibly spun.

Remaining silent and speaking at the right time is a great challenge to us all, because many of us have probably discussed all these discrepancies at home or in social settings, but failed to speak at the important moments. These points begin to fill more space in our daily life, which illustrates that our divine universal core emerges with increasing frequency, although we have not yet understood it in its entirety.

If we now allow ourselves to declare a new goal by simply assigning our previous goals a different value, we can begin with great determination to change this world in favor of peace, love and life in a way that serves us.

Everything on One Card

Big changes often require big decisions. Big decisions require a great deal of courage. The willingness to put everything on one card is a key characteristic of determination. Massive determination can also absolutely stem from the desperate attempt to FINALLY change something, because it is subconsciously clear that it is otherwise too late in one sense or another. Suicide bombers are an extreme negative example of this kind of determination. They put everything on one card. They end their own life and that of many others in the misguided belief, they are earning themselves access to heaven. We could be experiencing heaven on earth and don't have to either murder, or exploit, or do anything we think we have to do, in order to physically or mentally survive.

Behind every great vision is a strong image. A strong image brings trust with it. Trust in oneself and in life bears the possibility to solve all problems we find ourselves facing. This way we create real prosperity. True inner and outer wealth springs from the entirety of all of our parts. These parts make themselves known to us by way of our habits. Our previously negative habits invite us to take them home with great determination. They invite us to recognize them as what they are really meant for. The power bestowed upon us by unlimited trust in ourselves is the interconnection of all our parts to a single unit that acts in our intention – the divine experience to be one with everything. True freedom and independence come along with the insight, that we are connected to everything and therefore dependent on and responsible for everything.

Free Will

It is our choice whether we want to keep living in our scarcity-based thinking that, without our awareness, automatically accompanies our misinterpretation of success. This simply means that we will not retrieve all of our inner parts and thus will not consciously experience our divine universal origin, let alone live it. OR we can choose to enter into abundance-based thinking. This, by contrast, means that we retrieve every one of our inner parts and fully return to our divine universal oneness. We are all called upon to choose this inner unity and the divine, so that we may finally demonstrate on this earth what we came here for. True self-determination and freedom are the result, and true original and unconditional love accompanies them. Then we live our true selves and fully express our contribution to this world.

Miracles

If we are waiting for a miracle, I can lend us hope, for as soon as we act decisively based on this new awareness, more and more miracles will appear in our lives. Once we love ourselves entirely and completely, we ourselves will become the miracles we were born to be. In the final analysis, to love oneself means to recognize and express the whole and divine bundle within us. Miracles are the natural result of applying our nature and our origin. We have access to these miracles, when we find the trust and the courage to live and apply the universal rules of which everyone is a part.

This is only the beginning of something that we can merely guess at. Our determination can open the gates to our true nature. Then we can become the success, that we were meant to be from the beginning.

11. Perseverance

Perseverance is the incessant work on our trust and an essential part of success. No goal gets realized without perseverance. The foundation of perseverance is our will which, paired with desire, develops an irresistible pull in direction of the dream, thus causing ideas and goals to form.

People with perseverance can at times occur as egotistical. Due to a lack of consciousness we have forgotten how to express perseverance harmoniously with our surrounding.
An extremely authoritarian style of leadership was standard practice for many centuries. Values and goals that often had nothing to do with peace and love were upheld with absolute perseverance. But our development in the past 100 years has been quite positive in this respect, even though they contained two world wars. The Second World War also showed dramatically the consequence of perseverance, when it is not used for good. But we shouldn't stop here, because as you are reading this, violence and atrocities are taking place somewhere on this planet, because some human beings are holding on to their convictions with absolute perseverance. The perseverance to believe in certain norms and values is so powerful that, without reflection, it leads to all the suffering we encounter in the world. No less sad is the perseverance with which many people living in abundance avoid any feelings of responsibility for the poverty and exploitation in this world.

Yet perseverance can be destructive even on a small scale. Many people persevere and work countless hours, completely neglecting their health – all for the sake of their own safety and that of their families, and their desire for prosperity and happiness. With perseverance we put things into our bodies that can hardly be called food, while wondering why we keep getting sicker. We give drugs to animals and put them in food, then wonder why some substances have become ineffective while illnesses and allergies continue to spread. One would think that we meanwhile had heard of homeopathic principles, which could shed some light on this. The information in a substance whose traces are still physically measurable, as in homeopathic drugs, can have an effect on the body. But even the information in a substance that can no longer be physically measured can still produce effects. They work energetically, but more on a mental and emotional level. This is indeed a questionable approach, especially in light of the rising numbers of depression, burnout, cancer and "problem" kids or children with ADHS. If everything is energy, which quantum physics confirms more each day, than everything influences everything beyond the physical boundaries.

The perseverance to believe in competition quickly turns couples into competitors. They reenact on the small scale as separations and divorces what happens on the large scale as wars. It is no different among siblings. Add to that, the perseverant context of parenting, by which children must obey – which was and still is sometimes enforced via physical or verbal violence. We are persistent in trivializing numbers, data and facts of current manifestations of inhumanity by comparing them with those of the past, or even ignoring them. Our perseverance leads us to teaching and grading things in schools, that do not contribute to creating a foundation for interpersonal cooperation in daily life. Instead we teach numbers, data and facts from the past, but without correlating them to the present. And then we wonder why we're dealing with increasingly extreme forms of inattention, negligence towards life, things and people, as well as violence and destruction. This is, however, a logical result when we fail to teach which misguided values result in which consequences, or how power hunger develops in misunderstood people, so that they bully families, friends, classmates, teachers or colleagues in their daily environment, or influence entire nations if not the fate of the entire world on a global level. This selfish behavior rises also out of a misunderstanding. Somebody who is searching itself crosses the borders gladly, but most time the borders of others. Therefore, we are mostly all on our big quest to find ourselves, it is not surprising, that our common definition of success leads us to such an amount of selfish people and behaviors. Until today they were unable to experience a „healthy" self-empowerment. Therefore, they seek to express power through different channels, usually by dominating others. Under our current definition of success all that is "normal", although there is nothing natural about it.

Normal and natural

Perseverance as described in the last paragraph brings forth this world we call "normal". In the word itself we already can see an important factor – the norm. Norms are determined by people in order to make something easier to understand, compare and prove and to establish a guideline. Those norms are based on conditional love with its resulting thoughts, our beliefs and our actions.

Unconditional divine love, which is mentioned in our religions - but was never fully understood and thus diminished - is, what you could call "natural". Herein we find the word "nature". It is our nature to be kind, helpful and peaceful in our interactions with each other. But our belief that scarcity and separation exist, still misleading us into living in a way that can hardly be considered our natural state. Often, we don't even acknowledge it, because until now it has been unthinkable to view ourselves as divine, powerful and eternal. This is actually tantamount to blasphemy.

In spite of all this, it is nonetheless our nature, and it can bring us solutions to our challenges, if we are ready to truly acknowledge our light and let it shine. In our true nature as a part of the holy divine there is all what we are longing for. All the norms are included which would make it much easier to really understand, compare and prove. It would be normal to express the guideline, which is within all of us all the time, by our daily actions.

Prerequisites for Perseverance

Perseverance is based on the characteristics of success, which are discussed here in individual chapters. We have been using these characteristics the entire time – they merely require a new focus or a new superordinate value, so that all the resulting values, thoughts, objectives and actions can automatically be adjusted. Until now we just didn't realize that this superordinate instance of divinity and unconditional love needs to occupy a complete different space. Once we are able to do that, we can use the cascade of success to our best knowledge and for the benefit of everything that exists on this planet.

Emotional Pain Eraser

Perseverance always pays off in the end. The most important payoff is the knowledge, that each alleged failure carries in it the seed of future success and of our vocation and destiny. Very few people use the pain of a defeat in order to carry on. These people have learned to actively seek the positive in life and what there is to recognize from it. In pain we have the opportunity to know ourselves. Though, what's interesting is, that as soon as we evaluate the painful situation differently, the pain instantly disappears. The crisis becomes an opportunity.

The Consequences of a Lack of Perseverance

The consequences can be observed everywhere but so far have gone quite unnoticed. Our inability to clearly define what we want, goes hand in hand with great procrastination. It puts comfort above any need for change, no matter how direly needed it may be. It does not seem important to acquire more knowledge in order to get closer to the goal of peace and health. Instead we seem to misuse our perseverance for the enjoyment and expansion of our comfort zone. The truly relevant goals are treated with indecisiveness and "postponitis". A certain indifference and perceived helplessness as we know it from the problems in the world lead to lame compromises. As a result, the status quo is maintained or improved at the expense of the weaker parts in and around us. Accusations and a weak sense of responsibility lead us to claim, that they are responsible for the situation themselves. Our own part in it is deliberately overlooked, leading to a subconscious weakness and powerlessness with oneself and circumstances. The result is a weak desire, at best, to change anything; we simply give up at various junctures, or demonstrate strong resistance against concrete plans for change. Wishing replaces the will, underlining the compromises. Widespread scarcity-based thinking ensues, although there is plenty of wealth. We look for answers in areas that aren't even related to the root of the problem.

The Pitfalls of Perseverance

Many people are so trapped in their negative thinking that they wouldn't even recognize a chance or an opportunity if it bit them on the nose. On the contrary, they would scream and flail and smash it with a shoe because they don't recognize it as such. They experience it as bad, evil and destructive. In this way, they persistently serve their inner fears and negative experiences that have, until now, taught them something different.

Here an incisive example:
A woman had too little money and no job. Her friend offered to help; she would have liked to just give her a little money but the woman refused it. She didn't want to simply be given money, but to earn it, which is laudable. So they agreed, that she would

help her friend with a project and get paid for it. But the woman hardly showed up for work, so her friend asked her why she didn't work persistently on the project. She also asked her how much money she would need to make ends meet and the answer surprised her. The woman would have needed merely 2 hours, 5 days a week, to easily cover her needs. She failed to see the opportunity in that agreement. The gift of that relatively simple work, that she also enjoyed, was hidden because of her misconception. She didn't recognize the wealth she could have created herself, because she lacked the perception for it. Her poverty- and scarcity-based thinking had impacted her too greatly.

If we look at this theory in regard to the false definition and misinterpretation of success, it is quite likely that people would react to an enormous chance for true change on earth just like the woman in this story. We should be very clear about the fact, that a part of us has already unconsciously represented those useless patterns of thought, speech and/or behavior with perseverance "par excellence" our entire life long. Until now, this happens with such mastery that, we haven't even been able to notice it.

The Courage to Persevere

Courage is to face a fear and STILL accept the challenge even though we are afraid. Many people are waiting their entire life for THEIR chance in life. In the end they bitterly declare, "I never had a chance". It's like waiting your entire life for a four-leaf clover and disregarding the gift of all the three-leaf clovers. But the truth is: the only chance we can really count on is the one we create ourselves. It is said for good reason that luck is what happens when preparation meets opportunity. This means to prepare for what is important to us, so that we can act the way we want in the right moment.
The greatest desire of a human being seems to be the desire to

really be ourselves. All the areas like career, intimate relationship, family, sexuality, friends and whatever else is important, support us in finding our true self-expression. It takes all of our perseverance to establish this desire in life as an experience and to satisfy it.

Each time we persistently indulge in fear, we separate ourselves perseveringly from ourselves, who we really are, and what really matters to us, as well as automatically from the external equivalent inside another person and in our environment. With that, we persistently deny ourselves the perception of the world the way it could be. We unconsciously push away all that wealth, material or immaterial, in us or around us, and we destroy it, because we don't recognize it as wealth. This wealth lays far beyond what we currently define as wealth. One of the most important preparations for luck is to reflect and change, so that we can even see opportunities as chances in the first place. Right now, we have a unique opportunity and chance to change the world and turn it into what we want it to be – a peaceful and wonderful place. Are we going to take advantage of that chance?

The Solution Lay Within

The perseverance of our deepest universal origin is a most impressive thing. No matter how bad it gets for the individual, in our environment or on earth, love always finds a way to express itself and it can't be stopped. It is everywhere and spreading in everything that surrounds us. Even our most negative feelings are an expression of love; love that is misinterpreted and misunderstood. Fundamentally, love is omnipresent. It is like the plants that can't be permanently held back by asphalt, concrete walls or any other artificial barrier. If we allow nature to follow its path, it will always win in the end. And herein lay our chance and solution. If we allow our own true nature to arise, the things that don't serve us will give way of their own accord. The natural state of being of every human can lead to new standards that serve and are in harmony with our nature, and that are no longer opposed to our divine universal origin. We are on the verge of ringing in our own renaturation as human and divine universal being.

The knowledge of the universal order is anchored in all of us – it is part of our nature. The ethics of our soul is the authority that wants to make the universal order our new standard. Then we shall apply perseverance paired with love, respect, understanding and empathy to create an attraction and a pull, so that norm and nature can unite as one. It is then an urge rather than a must to be true to our goals and ourselves. This in turn creates even more attraction and a high level of trust. We have been looking for this trust for a long time on the outside, yet can it only be found within us. Here the true root of self-confidence reveals itself. If we are to experience fulfillment in all areas of life and peace on earth, it is imperative that we use the characteristic of perseverance purposefully – for our natural state and not for the existing norm. When we truly understand – not only with the intellect, but also with the nature of our heart – we change everything.

THERE IS NO SUBSTITUTE FOR PERSEVERANCE!

12. The Power of Community

Now we come to the part of this book that illustrates how important the environment and other people are. Among other things, we will learn how the power of change can arise from organized and intelligently applied knowledge. Success – no matter how it is defined – is not possible without other people. The advantages of community are obvious. The knowledge, experience and the energy of all involved are available and can be accessed. Generally speaking, communities have the best results, when all members are willing and able to support each other without reservation and in harmony. This happens, however, only in the rarest of cases. This operating principle is mainly known under the term success groups or mastermind groups.

Mastermind Groups

A German web article written by Andreas Mose offers the following explanation: *"The first mention of mastermind groups in success literature occurred in Napoleon Hill's book "Think and Grow Rich", which is also where the term mastermind group was coined. Hill knew of them from many of the 500 self-made millionaires that he interviewed for his book between 1908 and 1928... At the time, they often consisted of an army of the best advisors and experts on certain topics, among other great thinkers... Today we refer to a group of likeminded people who are independent of each other yet support each other in reaching their individual goals... The participants must be hungry for success and continuously raise their demands of themselves and others for these groups to unfold their full effect.* **At the same time, it requires, despite a healthy self-awareness, maintaining great openness and the willingness to continuously question oneself***... Another very important point is that participants should have similar values. Even though some friction is healthy, it makes no sense if one's own moral* *compass points in a completely different direction than those of the others..."*

In honest examination, we can see that we collectively represent a single great mastermind group, embodying the underlying hierarchal structures of our society that drive the clockwork of success. When we look honestly, we can recognize the unconscious "hamster-wheel clockwork" with its multitude of different "hamster-wheel cogs". As a quid pro quo, the sentence in bold print shows what failed to appear. We have misinterpreted self-awareness until now, and therefore this principle was employed by success and power-hungry people to their own ends, with self-confidence but no real self-awareness.

Mastermind groups are omnipresent, we are just not aware of this because we have rooted them mainly in the context of success and business. Mastermind groups include parents, families, clubs, churches, schools, colleges, parties and any group of people with the same basic convictions or similar values that are joining forces. The religious fanatics and warmongers on this planet use this principle as well. Everybody uses this principle completely subconsciously.
And once more again: With few exceptions, the entire world upholds similar values, which are all based on what we previously call success and failure!

Mastermind

Mastermind is taken literally "the mind of a master". In a spiritual or religious context God is also considered as master. Seen from this angle, the previous statements may begin to become clearer and gain a new meaning. If we are all part of a divine universal origin it would explain, why we, while lacking true awareness, are unknowingly connected through this mastermind or spirit. The eternal universal spirit is a main source of power, if not even THE main source of power. Any time two or more people join in harmony and work on a specific goal, they are able to include, through this joining, the mental storehouse of the universe. It is precisely those energies that a genius or person like Gandhi turns to. Our bible mentions this with the following words: *"For where two or three are gathered together in my name, there am I in the midst of them."* (Matthew 18:20) It is the energy which was buried and now comes to light again as soon as we transform our vulnerabilities and misinterpretations into potentials.

It is time to include a concrete definition of mastermind the way I understand it. It is based on the statement „all is one" and therefore the realization that everything is energy. "Mastermind is the coordination of effort and knowledge between two or more energies, that combine in harmony and equilibrium to reach a concrete common objective." Energy is meant here in the sense, that it includes any inner or external structure of oneself, of other beings, as well as everything that exists. In the context of our self it is the coordination of our own inner parts. This spirit inhabits all energy, not just humans, but also animals, plants, water, rock, earth, etc. - just everything that exists. It is important to realize that we have been connected and allied with this energy on the inside and the outside the entire time; but we misused this connection out of lack of knowledge and awareness. We were not aware of the community with all that exists.

Community

The word community contains in German two words: the word "common" and „create". According to Wikipedia, common originally means: "a quality which is owned jointly by multiple people". In this context it becomes clear that all beings, simply everything existing on this planet, have one thing in common: the subconscious and often not yet acknowledged divine universal origin. The German word for community reflects in the meaning what is our chance: that which commonly exists could be used constructively to create something together.

Without mastermind we cannot achieve big goals. For the individual, a big goal could be reviving an intimate relationship, finding a completely new way to deal with their children, or living one's own true expression. For the community of people, it could be to create an ecumenism that spans the entire world, or to create overall contexts in global economics that have the same goal: the expression of our common origin. So far all big goals have been set inside our materialistic understanding of success, which inevitably led to what we see today, since it only represents a small part of the whole truth about us.

"Everything has two sides, but we don't get it until we recognize the third side!" –Anonymous

Success as we have known it until now has always expressed the same old, generally opposing sides. The component that allows us to see the third side was previously inaccessible because it is rooted in what we thought was impossible. Self-AWAREness was used to a very small extent. When two or more people or inner parts align with each other in harmony on a certain thing, they create a potential for attraction. This is the psychic component of Mastermind. The special thing about it is, that when a group of people or inner parts connect and work in harmony, the energy resulting from the sum of all of them is available to each one individually.

It's important to understand this for two reasons. When an individual finds peace with themselves and their inner parts, and pursues for example with their partner or children a common goal, then all involved have access to the abilities and insight of the person who is already at peace with themselves. To this end it is worthwhile to get over our past hurts, which are ultimately co-responsible for disharmony. Herein we may find the origin of Gandhi's quote *"Be the change you want to see in the world."*

If ever more and more people are in harmony with themselves and collectively pursue, for instance, the goal of making their contribution to a world of peace and harmony, each of them is connected to the resources of this entire group that is aligned in harmony; and beyond that with the divine providence, of which we heard in Goethe's poem on commitment.

Effects of Internally and Externally Harmonious Communities

People take on the habit and power of thought of those, they are connected to in harmony. Harmony attracts harmony and more and more groups can form a bigger group as long as a common large-scale goal exists.
Gandhi, for example, was one of the most powerful people of his time in regard to power of change, because he was able to unite several million people in harmony under a clearly defined goal. That is a miracle considering that, at times, it seems impossible to even temporarily unite just two people in harmony. Harmony arises when two or more people have a burning desire for a common goal. Once this fire is strong enough, those people will overcome their own limits and the boundaries around them. In light of what presently surrounds us, it would be a good idea for us humans to become aware of ourselves and recognize the power of our universal origin, so that we can collectively create what the majority of us desire and which automatically averts what we don't want, but which seems to perpetually loom over our heads.

True power is primarily power over ourselves. It is based on abundance and unconditional love, whose constructive use includes love, esteem and respect of all living beings and all that exists. Power as a result of selfish and egotistic behavior is based on fear and scarcity and what we previously knew as success. Selfish in this context means the search for our own true self. Subconsciously we all contributed our part in the human community, so that we may reach this point in human history where we can recognize ourselves, if we so choose. Fear and misunderstood power have predominated long enough on this planet.

We are talking about a new understanding of power: power through attraction, acceptance, love and peace, and about co-existence with each other and everything – the components of the ethics of our soul – our natural need. The main characteristics of this are a much flatter hierarchy, team thinking instead of competitive thinking, recognizing potential, free development and creativity, free reign to reach defined goals – this potential is found in all of us and is governed by the ethics of the soul. This precipitates more motivation and courage, independence and creativity as well as self-confidence, personal responsibility and recognition. Unconditional love, our divine connection and the insight into ourselves, bring those traits with it as qualities and habits automatically. Once we are consciously connected, it becomes necessary to contribute in this sense. A vision and a bigger picture of the goal serve as guiding star. Co-ordination arises in harmony and equilibrium, in order to reach this goal that is deeply anchored.

Harmony

The etymology of the word harmony includes the Indo-Germanic syllable "ar" or "har", which means *"combining of opposites to a whole"*. Harmony can hardly arise as long as we don't realize how everything is interconnected and we unite the opposites to a whole.

"There are no great discoveries and advances as long as there is an unhappy child on earth"
Albert Einstein

Unhappiness means disharmony. Einstein already saw the important and essential part. This short quote demonstrates what we have touched on in many sections of this book: the fact, that we all bear responsibility for the misery in this world. With that, however, we also have the power to change in our hands, if we choose to direct all our knowledge and actions toward unconditional peace, health, love and the best result for all involved.

Each of us, however, also has another inner level of correspondence. Figuratively speaking, children are synonymous with dreams - lifelong dreams. The way we deal with children and being childlike, as well as the associated external persuasions, demonstrates, how we deal with our divine dreams, wishes and desires internally. This is because our surroundings could not allow these wishes due to the rules and norms of our previous thinking of success. Most of us still deal with our truly vital dreams of love, peace, health and true community in the same way – the way we learned to. As long as there are any unhappy children out there, it points to unhappiness, or the disharmony of our seemingly opposite parts within ourselves, and with that to our unawareness of ourselves. Unhappiness means the realization that previously lived goals don't coincide with the overall goal: TO BE YOURSELF.

When we all are ourselves, it becomes impossible for there to be an unhappy child on earth, because we are then living and expressing our true divine origin. Unconditionality results automatically. When all people are themselves, their mutual connection – through and with the Great Spirit that inhabits everything – causes everything necessary to also be done on the outside, so that peace and harmony can arise and endure.

It always takes at least two for war, but for peace it only takes one: the one, who is the first to stop with the war.

Community begins with *"love your neighbor AS YOURSELF!"*
As long as there are unrecognized parts of ourselves, this occurs as a back and forth between what was previously considered love and the original divine and universal kind of love. It is the

alternating between normality and flow. Normality, however, is not what is natural. What is natural is self-awareness, love and flow. Normality is mediocrity. Mediocrity that was fully misunderstood. Living a happy medium does not mean to live in mediocrity. A happy medium means to enjoy, celebrate and live the entire abundance and glory of our own being and origin from the flow of our own internal center.

Applied Knowledge is Wisdom

We practice the application of our knowledge throughout our entire lives. Subconsciously, however, much was based on scarcity and fear, and was applied automatically. We have always been at work on transforming our knowledge into wisdom through actions. We simply were missing the unknown X, which can join together the seemingly irreconcilable and senseless into a great general purpose, while indeed making possible the best result for all involved.
Now, we need only recognize the following: knowledge based on abundance and love becomes, when applied, positive wisdom. Knowledge based on scarcity and fear becomes, when applied, negative wisdom. Under the previous interpretation of success, many results appeared as success, when in fact they showed negative consequences in the overall context. So they are still negative wisdom - in regard to our goals of love, health and peace - and thus ill success, because the awareness of the correlation was missing.

Our knowledge of facts of history, of time and of science is dualistic; there are thesis and antithesis, depending on the point of view and surroundings of the creator of the thesis. Only the great unknown X can shed light on that mystery. This unknown X brings thesis and antithesis together. It is capable of creating reconciliation from the seemingly irreconcilable. This great unknown X is the boundless divine universal spirit and its expression through unconditional love – our true self-awareness. The boundless spirit is never wrong because it inhabits everything and everything arises from it.

The Quantum Leap

The quantum leap for humanity means to maintain the state of connectedness to divine universal love by becoming, being and staying present to the true self.

According to the German Duden *a quantum leap can be defined on one hand as the sudden transition of a microphysical system from one quantum state to another, or a progress made possible by a new idea, discovery, invention, insight, etc., which causes a dramatic level of development in a very short time span.*

If we examine the first point, we can apply this descriptive model as follows: our own inside = microphysical system, is transposed from the quantum state of scarcity and fear to the quantum state of abundance and love = self-awareness of our divine origin. Where the second part is concerned, the insights and perceptions we have read can help us to remember ourselves and which make that quantum leap possible. This reminiscence can massively further the individual within a very short time.

This applies also on larger scales when people join together in this love and self-awareness. Many individual groups join together around the world with the goal of creating peace on earth. These people believe in harmony and live it themselves more and more to the extent, that their current environments allow it. They connect and ally themselves and their dreams. They convert these goals into plans and actions. It is possible to cause a quantum leap for humanity in the direction of true self-awareness, love and peace on earth. The new definition of success would make that progress possible, which in turn would cause a dramatic level of development in a very short time span. The ethics of our soul have been there all the time to show us the way – the way to divine order and harmony. We just didn't understand how the true image of humanity and all that exists can be made visible by looking at that symbolic photonegative. In the time ahead we not only have the opportunity to recognize and create newly the image of humanity and life, but also the possibility, to make it into an entire movie with all sorts of special effects – a marvel of divine universal self-expression.

13. Union – A little different Meaning of Sexuality

We are born with sexual desire. Sex drive is something very natural, an irresistible force and a primal power – something that even children possess. The drive for sexual union in human beings has its absolute legitimacy, but this too has been misunderstood, just like our self-awareness, love, success and many, many other things. Sexual union fundamentally represents a completely different kind of union: the union which we have completely forgotten, and which we are now allowed to primordially recall. This misunderstanding is a relevant, yet so far completely overlooked factor in our success. The expansions of perception in this chapter show us the way to endless joy and happiness. The knowledge in this chapter has the power to appease the metaphorical void or black hole of our existential fears that arise when our previous values are questioned. In this chapter we find out, what can fill this void with possibility. Happiness and integral success are possible for each of us on a daily basis and on a global level for all of us, if we dare to change our understanding of success and our worldview. In this chapter we will explore why, and what this primordial force is really all about.

The word "sexual" and with it sexuality and everything related to it also fell prey to a misperception, and are thus primarily used in the sense of physical sexuality. At the German Wikipedia you can find the following wording: *"In a broader sense, sexuality refers to the entirety of life manifestations, behaviors, feelings and interactions of living beings in regard to their gender."* As we can see, sexuality encompasses much more than just sexual intercourse and the related topics. Here we are also conditioned too restrictively.

"Gender" is also not what we generally interpret it to be: the original definition of the word includes *"kind, sort, genus,"* and *"type or class"*. In the German Duden we can find: *"what pounds in the same direction."* Gender is an expression of our divine universal origin.

The saying *"the apple doesn't fall far from the tree"* finds its true origin here. Those of us, that are aware that they are divine beings express that and pass it on. Those that are unaware will express that unawareness and pass that on. Our "gender" is our divine universal origin. With that our opening sentence could read as follows:

We are born with the desire to express our true provenance. This drive is something very natural, an irresistible force and a primal power – something that even children possess. The drive to be one with oneself and all that is has its absolute legitimacy, but this too has been misunderstood, just like our self-awareness, love, success and many, many other things.

The manner and entirety of life manifestations, behaviors, feelings and interactions reveal whether an awareness of the „true gender" as divine being is present. Sexual energy demonstrates to what extent we are united with ourselves, accept ourselves and live according to that. Our original primal power can be guided and used to the extent, that our physical sexuality can be guided and used. If we use it in our best interest, we use it in the best interest of everybody around us. If we don't, misunderstandings begin to show up, leading to that which we will explore on the following pages.

Force and Power

Let us more closely examine the word "force" from "primal force". It stands out that force has a very negative connotation in our use of language: it is viewed as synonymous with *"power that abuses or destroys"*. The word power comes from the Latin *"potentia"*. The word potency, however, is found in completely different contexts in our use of language. One hand, we have dilution in homeopathic medicine, which is classified in potencies, and secondly in male sexuality as the ability to have an erection. We also find the term in mathematics. Obviously, however, potency or "potentia" actually means something different than what we are defining it as. One might think that it refers to the basic principle of power over something completely different. At Wikipedia the following wording about „force" can be found: *"Force is characterized as actions, processes and social contexts, in which or through which people, animals or objects are influenced, changed or damaged. This means the ability to act in a way that affects the inner or essential core of a situation or structure."*

When we combine the divine universal energy of unconditional love, with that core, which affects the entire inner structure of all of us, we realize that we would maybe influence or change but never damage. It appears, that the use of sexuality in the abuse of power is equally rooted in the misunderstanding that we find in the duality of fear and/or love. Our lack of understanding of awareness turned sexuality into the cause of boredom, misunderstandings, frustration and apathy in so many bedrooms. Moreover, sexuality has been reduced to so much less than it could be by skewed thoughts and belief systems. Meanwhile it is being almost completely drained of purpose, and unfortunately all too often also perverted. It has become one of the great evils of our time. I don't think it is necessary to go into depth on the many examples of derailed expressions of sexuality. We encounter them daily in great diversity.

Loss of Feminine Sexual Power

Over a long period of time, women have forfeited their knowledge of their original sexual power, which is linked to intuition. Often they were abused, tortured and killed in connection with exactly that inexplicable primal force, that lay far beyond the physical expression of sexuality. For a long time, women were made to deny themselves simply because they saw and approached things differently than men. In some areas on this planet, rape and violence against women and girls is seen as normal, as the media remind us on a regular basis. This image was mercilessly forced upon us over many eras until we forgot who we are inside of that sexuality, forgot what it is really about, and what powers lay dormant within us. Generations later, these negative energies still show their aftereffects, even though this violence and brutality is, at least in the Western world, much less present today.

We unlearned how to listen to this voice of intuition and forgot everything connected with it. Consequently, the balance between man and woman and the expression of sexuality were inevitably altered. This is how it probably was possible that men as well as women forget what sexuality is and can truly represent; thus we now live inside of a predominantly male-dominated image of sexuality. Intuition is the connection to what is partially impossible to be put into words. Our world, however, demands numbers, data and facts. Thus the inexplicable is often not expressed, and we no longer trust our own guidance, also in questions of sexuality. The attribute of female guidance in men as well as women is, however, very important for a change in our sexuality, as well as the change of everything else. Sexuality is like a stream. You can build dams and control it; however, at some point the dam will break if it is not utilized with creativity and purpose, but used destructively. It will find alternate forms of expression in order to compensate, as we all too often experience.

Yin and Yang

How do these manifestations come to be? To the masculine is metaphorically attributed the day, light, action and the giving. To the feminine is metaphorically attributed night, darkness, quiet and receiving. Positive habits can metaphorically be assigned to the day, thus the masculine in us. Negative habits – which, as we already explored, are but a misunderstanding of our potentials – and fear are assigned to the night, which is attributed to the feminine in us. It's no surprise, then, that the feminine is not in harmony with the masculine. Nobody wants to have those perceived negative habits and experience that emotional night (darkness), which in turn causes a permanent rejection of those characteristics and of feminine power. This can be explained by the fact, that the feminine itself seems to have forgotten the feminine for millennia. Women experienced the receiving characteristic in a very unhealthy way. They experienced the receiving of external circumstances to the point of self-abandonment and they were neither aware of themselves, nor accepted or took themselves seriously, because they were forbidden to do so. The more women lost their feminine aspects, the less they were able to pass them on through the birth and upbringing of children. An ever-growing imbalance was created, along with a surplus of the masculine principle. Masculine here does not just mean masculine on the outside, but also the inner masculinity inherent in each woman and man, which appears in many forms through all our actions. Both women and men have forgotten their true expression, which lay slumbering in each of us.

This inner guidance or intuition continually invites us to accept this lost and forgotten power, so that the balance can finally be restored. The masculine and feminine aspects, regardless of whether in a man or a woman, want to be in balance. Harmony and balance then bring the desired healing. This wish for unification is deeply rooted, however the chosen expression through sexuality alone is not expedient and just a small partial aspect of true union. The result is, that we don't recognize the misunderstanding and seek on the outside what is missing on the inside.
The masculine part is the force within us, that gives space to

feminine guidance and intuition, so that vigorous and purposeful action can occur. Intuition is the feminine part within us, that steers the energy and creative force onto the right track and causes deep purpose and fulfillment in life.

Dissatisfying Sex

Even in relationships lived with love this masculine-dominated image of sexuality fails to cause true satisfaction in its ramifications. There are many humans who don't quite know what they really desire or what they want. Often there may merely exist a vague feeling of "different" or "not like that". But this perception in no way means that those would dare to express this; for often there is no reference available for what is missing, so the "different" is entirely intangible. "Not like that" expresses the search for harmony between body, mind and soul in sexuality. However, often only the body is considered. Women are often highly sensitive and actually perceive our normal manner of sexuality as something akin to abuse – the abuse of themselves. This misunderstanding tends to create dissatisfaction, or at times "boredom" in their love life, which then demands ever-increasing abstinence on one hand or ever increasing stimulation on the other hand. The desire for sexual union can be so great and irresistible, that people will voluntarily risk life and reputation for it.

And one thing more: On one side, more and more people demonstrate a growing readiness to appear naked or scantily clothed, and on the other side people who desperately want to capture and publicize this. This seems to be the fully misunderstood primal longing of the soul. We want to show ourselves the way we are and see the other the way they really are. We want to feel seen, loved and respected. But this primal longing relates more to the inner and not primarily to the exterior „nakedness". And one more point: This paragraph offers us in a figurative sense two incisive core statements with an important message. I will swap out a few words: Even in jobs experienced with happiness, this masculine-dominated image of life fails to cause real satisfaction in its ramifications. The desire for success can be so great and irresistible that people will voluntarily risk life and reputation for it.

Prerequisites for The New Path

Especially women are often very unfulfilled without ever really showing or expressing it noticeably. They often have little use for conventional sexuality. They are longing for openness and acceptance, to lose themselves in space and time and to drown in the void. This, however, requires the willingness to show ourselves up to our partner and to allow and experience whatever and wherever this desire leads to. This means to accept guidance, guidance that comes from within. We have to examine old habits, and walk the resulting new paths of action or lack of action with conscious control of old thoughts as well as impulses. Women are called upon to communicate and to indicate what this inner voice really wants from sexuality and during sex. Of course, there will be also men, who will retrieve themselves in this description, because they are also a union of male and female parts.

Intuition connects us with the power of our true sexuality. It takes primarily two things in order to grant listening to this inner guidance: trust and time. It requires time to feel and recognize what is really happening, and to get involved first and foremost with oneself, so as not to simply do what many people claim is the way sexuality works. Furthermore, it takes trust that the woman is ok with what she feels. The courage to recognize and change what is undesired is a basic requirement. The trust that her inner guidance will know the path out of the habitual sexuality is indispensable. Also in this so vital part of life it is revealed just how important intuition is, in the form of the tender voice of inner guidance as a direct line to the divine core. It is often merely a whisper that is periodically drowned in daily life.

If we take that last paragraph and replace "woman" with "human being" and "sexuality" with "life", we again get a higher-level equivalent: *Intuition connects us with the true power of our life. It takes primarily two things in order to grant listening to this inner guidance: trust and time. It requires time to feel and recognize what is really happening, and to get involved first and foremost with oneself so as not to simply do what many people claim is the way life works. Furthermore, it takes trust that a human being is ok with what they feel. The courage to recognize and change what is undesired is a basic requirement. The trust that the inner guidance will know the path out of the habitual life is indispensable.*

What If?

The path toward oneself contains a magnificent and unique sexuality, since it is the logical consequence of trusting oneself and one's own guidance. Sexuality performed with love has the potential to connect people newly with themselves and their innermost being. It even has the power to open the path to ourselves when we are very far from ourselves. Those who follow those small, delicate impulses and open up to them, are able to experience how interplay arises.

Those who don't experience the desired sexuality will often perceive a feeling of "that should feel different!" This leads to the conclusion, that there is a recollection of how sexuality and union are actually meant. A profound knowledge of when alignment is present and the higher self gets expressed, seems deeply anchored, and an insatiable desire arises to bring the exterior closer to the inside and not vice versa. A primordial treasure map inside of us seems to exist, that wants to guide us to the expression of our true self. It is time to acknowledge this map and follow it. Sexuality and love are the strongest incentives for that. It makes wounds heal faster, almost automatically, through which the true self can be discovered. The mere possession of sexual energy is of little use. But the desire to be oneself uses this sexual power. Sexual energy reaches its true power of deployment when progressively more self-love, self-knowledge and self-awareness are present. Sexuality inside of the most profound self-love is not exorbitantly used but creatively utilized – and not just during sex.

The true One

The permanent search for the one true love, or the love and relationship for life seems omnipresent and deeply rooted. It is curious that this topic is present to such a degree and serves as a core plot in fairy tales, movies, books, plays, operas, musicals, poems, etc. ... Many know this longing for the one true love deep inside themselves – a longing from not yet having found someone or something. But many remain disillusioned in what they are now – dissatisfied, unhappy, helpless and powerless. Countless unhappy relationships, skyrocketing divorce rates, as well as an increasing number of people who choose to live single, outline a path we don't yet understand. It seems as if many relationships are bogged down with both partners "blind" to their own needs, and thus to those of the other person as well. There is a reason for this longing for a fitting match. It might well be found in the need of both parties for a different mirror, in which they can recognize why they are both really in this world: their own primordial expressions of themselves.

Everything points toward the need for a different mirror for the next better version of our own self, without which the original version cannot be recognized and experienced, since we are missing reference experiences. Many couples have shackled each other – not each the other, but rather each themselves FOR the other, out of misinterpreted love. This misinterpreted love is based on a fear and scarcity-orientation, and ultimately the fear of the loss of safety, purpose and community. But in the moment when we give ourselves the freedom of wanting to find the answer to who we truly can be, we also give the same right and opportunity to the other person. On this path, not merely doors, but gates to ourselves open in a very short time. The partner exists that makes the potential visible, which is missing for our internal partnership and union. The recognition happens often in the same moment and both know *"That is what I have been waiting for my entire life!"* When both of these partners or souls find each other, it means growing side by side, enduring the other's mirror, allowing what is and loving it. It also does not necessarily have to result in a romantic relationship in the conventional sense. The point of this deep relationship is, regardless of how it is experienced, to recognize each other IN-DEPENDENTLY as that which each one is, in order to finally be oneself and experience that. Both have the chance to know themselves fully and completely by way of each of them developing the potentials the other already has, so that they can share with the world whatever self-expression they brought with them into this life.

Those who just wish to flee shall be forewarned. No matter where we flee to, we will always be confronted by ourselves and our innermost truths; for you cannot run from yourself. Those who keep silent out of fear to hurt or lose the other person is hurting or losing themselves, regardless whether it is the old or the new partner. Those who recognize and love themselves recognize the fears in themselves and in the other person that prevent both from changing. You can separate and still treat each other well, especially when there are common children, in which case it should be a duty. If the welfare of the latter is made the top most priority in the situation surrounding the separation, certain war-of-roses scenarios will rule themselves out on their own. The ethics of the soul will automatically lead one on the path to separation with love.

Deep love towards another person opens the heart and with it the gates to our self. But the positive behavior of being in love was until now in a sense connected to that person on the outside. We did not recognize that these were our own qualities that we can access at any time, independently of this other person outside of ourselves. We made ourselves dependent because we thought the other person was responsible for our own feelings and reactions. But the other person is not the cause. They show us the cause inside us, for their presence and behavior prompts us to reveal our true core on the outside and to allow this love. The inner unity grows progressively when we begin to feel from within ourselves that, for which we needed the partner. The new desire to be true to ourselves attracts the same on the outside, and becomes real as a consequence. Finally, this relationship can be experienced on the outside – the relationship, that seemed so impossible. The outside can now become the desired mirror of our own inside.

The Healing Relationship

"Love evidently retains the power to transform experiences made by unfavorable relationships, and to make the dried up sources of our creativity accessible for us again." Gerald Hüther

There is no room in a healing relationship for the illusion of safety, because it comes with claims of ownership, a desire to be in control and mutual sabotage. Conversely loyalty, friendship, reliability, space for individual freedom and authenticity are the pillars of a healing relationship. Freedom is not meant here in the sense of indiscriminate sex or free love, but of not wanting to control the other – not even by withholding one's own authentic truths out of fear of hurting or losing the other person, or simply just out of well-meaning. The space for the self-development of the other person would be curtailed as a result, and their further development impeded. But in actual fact one's own development would be thwarted.

A healing relationship signifies being clear that there are

projections – actions and situations that one does not like, but are perceived that way, because we pull on our victim/perpetrator filter, and that they have to be continuously questioned. That means to always first ask: what does this have to do with me? Especially when it hurts the most. This often goes hand in hand with very deep emotions and requires a lot of integrity and sensitivity. It is important to accept each other as teacher or coach, to learn how to admit, when we cover the other person in our own false perception, and to possibly be willing to accept help from precisely the person that appears to be the cause of our deep pain. Respect, true compassion and trust are the requirements for this.

Power plays (weakness and strength or being right and fault) have a continuously shrinking role in this relationship. This sort of relationship requires the courage to jump over one's shadow a hundred if not a thousand times, and to open one's heart again and again, even if we would prefer to run miles away or crawl under the next rock and never come out again. This means to show up ourselves – in our own time – with our pain and our faults, and to admit it all and place it all in this field of trust, knowing that neither the other nor oneself intends to cause harm, but only to experience the best outcome. This applies to the relationship with a partner on the outside, as well as the relationship to ourselves on the inside.

A Somewhat Different Approach

Sexuality and unification have one requirement, if we want to be catapulted onto the Cloud No. 9 of lust: self-awareness and self-love. When man and woman unite in the greatest possible harmony, they experience unity and oneness. Those who are in unison with their inner parts can through sexuality experience on the outside, what so many yearn for. I will more closely illustrate this "process" since this will be of great importance for our "picture of success" later on.

To keep it simple, I will call this energy in all of us the primordial sexual energy. The difference in experiencing sexuality is grandiose. This energy catapults us into worlds, we barely had access to until now. The difference can be most easily explained through the experience of what we call the climax. In the prevalent masculine-oriented sexuality – I call it this way, because action/doing is assigned to the masculine, which is in the foreground here – we work with a great deal of movement and action towards reaching the climax.

This is completely different in the original experience. In this manifestation of sexuality, feeling is fundamentally in the foreground rather than action. The partners explore each other's bodies, accompanied by the most tender of movements. The impulses as to where to go next come from the inside. Often a long tender foreplay takes place first. This foreplay is fueled by a deep desire to perceive and explore the other person and oneself. A delicate inner voice indicates whose turn it is with the tenderness. It is like a delicate ping-pong game of lust during which there are continuously new surprises, provided one is willing to expand and trust their perception. The union is tender and intense, but with little movement of the body. The body is less in motion, more so energy and the mind. The intellect is entirely geared toward feeling and allows us to perceive everything that happens. This causes energies to surge with continuously increasing intensity. Inside and outside are perceived simultaneously. Shaking and waves of extreme excitement repeatedly course through the body, which is carried on a bed of the tenderest energy. Jolts of energy are racing through the spine and flooding the body. The climax of the woman originates from a completely different epicenter. It also is not so much a climax, but an ecstatic state that simply sweeps one away. It is not an excited looking forward, but just an allowing of being washed over by these ecstatic waves, which can be noticed from afar - just like a gift. This state expands from the spine through the entire body and is more like an implosion than an explosion. It happens continuously in intervals. Several minutes can pass before this state subsides. It feels as if one were sensually reduced to one's sexual organ and as if every cell of the body sensed nothing but lust. These orgasmic states have women suddenly and automatically fall into rhythmic movements, which underline this process in a grandiose manner. This rhythm in turn excites the man who before simply surrendered to the inner voice and the lust. He experiences similar states as if infected by her energies. The highest bliss in the sexuality of a man seems to be attained in witnessing a woman filled with ecstasy. This experience nourishes and fulfills him, and leads him also into the highest ecstasy. His lust is her lust and vice versa – both are one. It is not uncommon that during a pause new waves of excitement arise which again wash over the body in orgasmic waves. This can last for hours. Many waves of lust can be passed through – ever swelling and subsiding. The inner guidance always knows what is next and when it is enough. It is simply the order of the day to follow it. This experience is marked by an incredibly strong physical and mental presence. Entirely different potentials of perception open up. What one feels cannot be put into words. One is simply FULFILLED!

Conclusion: This kind of sexual union does not need to be learned. It comes out of us, if we are self-aware and listen to our inner guidance and if we allow it to happen.

When we compare the common manner of sexuality with the manner of the one just described, you could say the act of love is simply reversed, however the result is not added but potentiated. Here potency shows up again, from the Latin "potentia" = power. In the commonly known manner of sexuality, there is first physical action in the foreground with the goal of an orgasm. When it is reached comes the resting phase, detumescence and for the man quite possibly falling asleep. But this is often when the woman just has the feeling of being warmed up. With the original sexual energy, it is exactly the other way around. In the beginning we enjoy feeling with little movement. Lust increasingly builds up and spreads through the body. With the climax, lust is automatically accompanied by rhythmic movement, which in the old manner we have to actively bring forth. To not allow this movement in that moment would be to block the path of that energy. This new kind of sexual energy does not mean we renounce movement and action. It occurs on its own, if the woman allows the path of her own feminine sexual energy and the man comes along and follows. Experiencing this kind of sexuality leaves both trembling. It takes both to completely new heights of lust and unsuspected depths of the current relationship. It is characterized by a great deal of attentiveness, attention, presence and the willingness to completely embark on each other. It is precisely this energy we can metaphorically utilize.

The Sexual Union

The sexual act seems to exists to remind us, what it would be like to be one with ourselves and our origin. Our spirit wants to show, what was meant for us and what is possible. How high our spirit swings and how much we express our genius, uniqueness and individuality depends to a significant degree with what level of sexuality and union – inside and out – we settle for. In our sex drive lay the key to great creative ability, individual uniqueness and genius in us all. Sexuality is the creative propulsion of all geniuses. This tells less about the frequency and more about the quality of the sexuality and with it the inner union. Here lay one of the deepest roots of our true self. Anyone who has ever experienced true love and has been propelled by it to maximum performance knows, that this love leaves a lasting impression in the soul. That impression never goes away. This quality springs from a different level. Even the mere memory of this love can produce peak performance in creativity. The deepest trust results from this profound connection to oneself, which wants to make us aware of the true scope of love.

Let us take a section of the description of sexuality above and apply exactly the creativity mentioned by "translating" what was written in the above paragraph about the original sexuality:

To keep it simple, I will call this energy in all of us the divine universal energy of life. The difference in experiencing life is grandiose. This energy catapults us into worlds we barely had access to until now. The difference can be most easily explained through the experience of what we call success. In the prevalent masculine-oriented manner to live – I call it this way, because action/doing is assigned to the masculine, which is in the foreground here – we work with a great deal of movement and action towards reaching success.

This is completely different in the original experience. In this manifestation of living, feeling (being) is fundamentally more in the foreground. The impulses as to where to go next come from the inside. This play of life is fueled by a deep desire to perceive and explore oneself, the other person, as well as life itself. A delicate voice indicates, when it is the masculine or the feminine aspect's turn with their life expression. It is like a delicate ping-pong game of life expression, during which there are ever-new surprises, provided one is willing to expand and trust their perception. It is like feeling one with oneself and with everything that is. Success is not an excited looking forward but just an allowing of being washed over by the universal events, which can be noticed from afar - just like a gift.

Conclusion: This kind of success does not need to be learned. It comes out of us if we are self-aware and listen to our inner guidance and allow it. When we compare the common manner of living with the one just described, you could say the act of life is simply reversed, however the result is not added but potentiated. This new kind of living does not mean we renounce DOING and ACTION. It occurs on its own. To not allow this DOING in that moment would be to block the path of life.

Success and Sexuality

We carry in us all the stimulants and motivators needed to reach a higher vibration in us. It is unnecessary to resort to negative and self-destructive stimulants like alcohol, drugs or other addictive substances or behaviors. There is no substitute for what the medicine cabinet of the body can deliver, when we are aware of our divine universal gender. We can then automatically resort to these resources.

A creative mind is only determined and propelled by the quality of the emotions. As we have seen, there are also other means to propel the mind, but none of them, not even in their sum, comes close to the power of sexual energy the way it is meant, through recognizing our true origin. Power from love is self-empowering and always has the best possible outcome for all in mind. It produces by proper utilization of the sexual impetus almost superhuman energy. Serenity, certainty and an unclouded faculty of discernment arise when self-love and sexual impetus unite. Sexual impetus is the desire driving us to finally become completely aware of our true gender, so that we can bring forth this wonderful union.

Is it surprising that there are so many aberrations and confusions, as well as violence and abnormality in the area of sexuality in that desperate search for the true "gender" of our divinity? Probably not. This awakening of awareness and the accompanying changes in personality occur through heart and emotion and not through the intellect. However, we most certainly and urgently need it to become, be and stay aware.

A Different Understanding of Open Love and Polyamory

Polyamory has also been reduced to mere physical love as a result of already established false definitions. It is abused in the sense of missing understanding and awareness of ourselves.

To live open love is a profound desire. But we have discovered that the love and self-awareness we were born with represent much more, than we are accustomed to experiencing. True love and the gift each one of us is, just want to be shared openly. Basically we just long to be able to love openly without misunderstandings, misjudgments and condemnation. This forgotten, denied and completely misunderstood part of us is longing to combine and unite itself with all souls, in love the way it is truly meant, with all its infinite expressions beyond physical sexual love. We just want to be able to love and trust. This part always focuses the good, the same divine provenance in the other, and wants to experience this relationship, which reflects its own relationship to the divine origin, as often as possible and preferably always. This union is what feels to us like "being home". It reminds us of how things were before we incarnated into this life. We primordially remember our origin.

The primary focus is not the physical union but the mental, energetic and spiritual union out of the awareness of ourselves and with it the awareness of everything around us.

The most important requirement for polyamory the way it is meant to be, is true and real self-awareness, self-consciousness and self-love. With this it becomes obvious how, when and with whom what kind of expression of relationship wants to be experienced. No matter which expression it is, it will be characterized by deep love, understanding, attention, respect and deep trust, for it reflects the same divine universal origin. With it we recognize ourselves.
Until now massive attraction between two people has been redirected into physicality, without questioning the cause of this attraction to another. Everyone that is meant to show us something about ourselves will send a strong signal of recognition through this sexual attraction. If we merely use it to slip into physical love, we will not recognize the actual gift.
Self-awareness and self-love bestow upon us automatically the

necessary distance to a person without renouncing love. We then know, which form and quality of a relationship we should experience with whom. This sexual energy is not something we do, but rather an expression of the divine energy when we are connected to our own origin. It is the state of being most connected with everything that exists, and where our masculine and feminine attributes are in harmony. The refocusing on our divine universal origin requires our full will, our full strength and, most importantly, our full commitment. We ourselves are the love of our lives in all our "sexually" united, aware and universal power. This is the longed-for intimate relationship meant for life, not as a single lifetime, but as an expression of life itself and with that for eternity.

It is up to us when we want to primordially remember. That is our FREE WILL that we have so often misunderstood. This PRIMORDIAL MEMORY is just the BEGINNING. The beginning of life the way it was originally meant. Genius, ecstatic, grandiose… simply life… simply love… simply heavenly.
PRIMEMBER – YOU ARE LOVE!!!

Summary and Essence

In order to fresh the remembering of the universal game rules, I would like to summarize the pri-minder characteristics aka the success characteristics. They show us, how we can find and use other, more meaningful and more expedient ways through true self-awareness and the knowledge that we have always been one with everything. In doing so, we transform the meaning of our lives, our worldview, and the course of history. Yes, it could be so easy, if we could allow us to expand our perception and experiences out of our universal roots. We just misunderstood who we truly are.

We don't need to learn anything new. We neither need to be more successful, nor to achieve anything else, except to remember that we are already one with everything. We have not recognized until now, that the inner change is our biggest challenge, because we just thought, the changes out there are in the foreground. This inner change will be the greatest challenge we have to deal with our entire life long and on earth. When the inner change is made, the rest will become Childs play considering to what we had to face with before.

In the **fear chapters** we heard that all fears originate in the fear of loss. Our misinterpretation led us to placing our focus on the fears of poverty, illness, death, being alone and futility, blocking our view of the solutions. We were not aware what we were actually so afraid of losing wealth, health, life, love and purpose. By shifting focus, the solutions are now within our grasp, since our entire way of thinking and acting can be completely reconsidered and reoriented.

Since the beginning of time, we humans have carried a burning **desire** for change on the one hand and continuity and security on the other. We live in an age of perfect means and confusing goals, as Albert Einstein already ascertained. The moment we shift our focus and bring the forgotten variable X on board, we can see that the burning desire for change in us can bless us with inner peace and peace on earth. Hope becomes conviction and certainty, because everything makes sense. With that, we can experience a greater level of continuity and security than ever before – the divine universal order and leadership within us, around us and through us. Trust in „God", as well as self-confidence and security in a community of like-minded people is the logical consequence.

On the topic of **trust** the following quote illustrates the results of our misunderstandings: *"On the debris of our despair we build our character"* (R.W. Emerson). Every person builds their character on the basis of what remains of their self-perception. Thus from a misunderstood self-confidence, a misunderstood self-awareness and in the end a "false" worldview had to emerge. Our respective life – a small fraction of what we truly are – stems from this perspective. We are the authors of the misunderstandings of our nowadays world. Our old truths have turned us into illiterates of life. Only when we unlearn these old truths, question them, examine them, and recognize them in true self-awareness, will we learn to read, understand and truly trust life and ourselves. The good news is that all of life is change. Therefore, the illiteracy of the 21st century can also be transformed.

The manner in which we speak to ourselves is crucial to our success. Anything imaginable, repeated over and over again, can be suggestion and can become **autosuggestion**.
This way of thinking causes us to assess our world as "right". Emotions are our „enthusiasm", for emotions are the expression of life. This determines our welfare and our woe. Anyone who knows themselves as a divine universal being also knows the responsibility regarding their „enthusiasm". True self-awareness recognizes that a different reality, and with it different circumstances can be conceived and brought about. For this

new reality, entirely new ways of thinking, feeling, speaking and acting will be adopted.

Anyone who gives expression to **wishes and desires,** through targeted actions, will be able to enjoy the fact that knowledge is power. Apparently until now we were missing the overall purposefulness independent of a material result, which led to the fact, that all of our knowledge and experience seemed useless with regard to our deepest desire for love, peace and health. Our human past along with all correlated experiences and all of our knowledge will only make sense, if we no longer forget and deny our spiritual past and instead recognize, integrate and most importantly, act on it.

When we look at all of our **knowledge**, we can realize, that we have a very strong intellect. But when we observe the condition of many people and the circumstances on earth, it is clear that we must have misunderstood something. Now, however, we are standing at the threshold of a new era, in which the divine essence is revealed and reason can slowly but surely be applied as reason. Our thinking becomes reason when we accept and live our divine universal origin. Our brain thinks. Our reason understands. This is possibly the beginning of the utilization of the unused portions of our brain. Then we will know what actions to take to create heaven inside ourselves and therefore on earth and experience it with all of our senses.

Fantasy or imagination is the switchman for our future successes. That which we have seen as intellect brought us to our fantasies, plans and the results we have to face today. Our imagination muscle has always been powerful – now, however, the HOW and WHY are decisive. What should we use our imagination and energy for? For fear or love? For blinders or expanded awareness? For complete health or illness? For intact relationships on ALL levels or for competition and conflict? For hell on earth or paradise on earth? Einstein once put it right on the money: *"We shall require a substantially new manner of thinking if mankind is to survive."* A new understanding of success would be the foundation that can give our imagination wings. Regardless of what area we wish to make progress in, we need a win-win between heart and intellect. We then give rise to a win-win of values and goals with tools and methods.

Success as we know it has until now been strongly linked with **Action**. This has led to a faster and faster turning of the rat race, leaving hardly any time to reflect, while rapidly spreading sense of futility. Until now the ultimate goal and the purpose of success was the result – generally as a materially measurable unit – that was intended to document "more of something", i.e. money, goods, etc. All ideas, planning processes, operating procedures and results were brought in line with this definition of the goal. Goethe understood our greatest challenge extremely well when he said, *"When compared with the ability to organize the work of a single day reasonably, everything else is child's play."* If the "more" and the entire process were aligned with the divine universal origin – the actual meaning of life – we could sustainably generate a plethora of love and positive energy, as well as peace, prosperity, health and growth. This world does not need to be saved, if we finally refrain from destroying it and preventing the possibility of self-healing of people as well as the entire environment. It is time to allow the flow of life and with it love, harmony, peace and health, and to enjoy with all senses that which was given to us – eternal life.

Everything we experienced in is stored and structured in our **subconscious**. This is the interface between us, all things and our divine truth. Since we don't see the world as it is, but as we see ourselves, a likeness is created of what we think and hold as truth internally. The conscious mind communicates with the subconscious, and through that with the superconscious. Our intuition is the dedicated line to this network and serves as a compass that wish to lead us to the miracles of life. The great source speaks to us always and wants to show us, how the world – in other words we – really are and could be. We have simply forgotten how to listen.

Self-awareness is an indispensable component of success and the first step toward change. Four crucial elements are necessary: courage, trust, openness and honesty. We need to trust ourselves and others in order to show ourselves as we truly are, and courage to allow this and to acknowledge completely new perspectives, as well as to question old ones. Similarly, we need openness in order to even believe in the possibility of a new way and a new worldview, and honesty along with the concession, that the old way has not led to the desired success. The term "self-awareness" has been misunderstood and originally means to be aware of one's own divine universal origin and to express that in one's being and actions. Only then does one recognize their true power and – more importantly – their responsibility. A compulsion to change the world arises, since the condition of the world causes emotional suffering, that will no longer be tolerated. Self-aware people do whatever is needed, wherever it is needed, and when it is needed. Success as we have lived it until now is not wrong, but simply a very small fraction of what is possible.

Without **determination** there would be no success. We apply this characteristic thousands of times each day automatically. One part of us represents the old, unquestioned standards and goals of our current worldview – which is in desperate need of a general overhaul – with great determination. Big changes often require big decisions and a great deal of courage. The decisive characteristic of strong determination is the willingness to stake everything on one card. This could definitely stem from the desperate attempt to finally change something, since it is subconsciously clear, that it is otherwise probably too late in one sense or another. If we are waiting for a miracle, there is hope, for as soon as we act decisively based on this new awareness, miracles will show up in our lives and we ourselves will become the miracles we were born to be. This same decisiveness can create a completely new worldview with new priorities and goals, inside of which profit receives a new meaning without being short-changed. It is merely probable, that we will recognize, create, maintain and most importantly, enjoy profit in other things beyond material riches.

Perseverance is the incessant work on our trust and an essential component of success. Without perseverance, a goal will not be realized. Due to a lack of awareness, our perseverance has brought about until now the world that we currently define as "normal". A certain indifference, along with perceived helplessness, leads to lame compromises that result in the preservation or improvement of the status quo at the expense of the "weaker" part of ourselves and of society. If we are to experience our fulfillment in all areas of life, as well as peace on earth, it is imperative that we apply perseverance sensibly – for the benefit of our natural, divine universal origin, instead of the current norm. Our will and our desire for change develops an irresistible pull in the direction of this dream. When we truly understand, we will change everything. THERE IS NO SUBSTITUTE FOR PERSEVERANCE!

The power of community has been underestimated until now. Mastermind groups are ubiquitous – we are simply not aware of them. Humanity as a whole is one gigantic mastermind group that defines and propels the wheelwork of success. Literally speaking, mastermind means "the spirit of the master"; the spirit that connects us all in harmony, when we allow it to do so. The new definition of success would allow us true progress. That would forward our development dramatically in a very short amount of time. It is possible to instigate a quantum leap for humanity in the direction of self-awareness, love, health and peace on earth. The ethics of our soul has been trying for a very long time to show us the way to divine universal order and harmony, which we together are called to restore. This is what „socialism", „fundamentalism" and „radicalism" actually mean in their purest, most loving and original form. We have simply never understood that, because we were missing the decisive „key" for any attempts at change.

The word "sexual" and, with it, **sexuality and union**, as well as everything correlated also fell victim to false perception. In a wider context, sexuality means the totality of life manifestations, behaviors, feelings and interactions between living beings in regard to their gender. In this way the word gains an entirely new fundamental meaning with new fundamental goals and ways. Gender is also not what we generally interpret it to be: the original definition of the word includes "kind, sort, genus," and "type or class". The demand for expression of our true gender – divinity – is innate. This impetus is something totally natural and an irresistible power, a primordial force that lives even within children. We have forfeited the knowledge of this primal "sexual" power and significance, which is interconnected with intuition.

The balance between man and woman, or more exactly between the male and female qualities within us, and the true definition and true expression of sexuality could no longer be handed down. It was necessarily forgotten that, at the core, it is not about physical union, but rather the mental, energetic and spiritual relationship to all that exists, and the awareness of our true selves and thus everything around us. We ourselves are the love of our life with our complete "sexually" united, aware and universal power. Success and life do not need to be learned. They come from within, if we listen - listen with self-awareness to ourselves and our inner guidance.

The True Identity

The misperceived longing for the love of our lives – the one true love or the "right" relationship – now brings me to the conclusion of the individual chapters. The following quote illustrates in very few words the understanding and misunderstanding we are fundamentally dealing with. I could not have expressed it more concisely.

"My deepest identity is the love of another soul... and this love is for me to protect, for otherwise I lose my identity, the meaning of life... to me, this is the greatest love on earth, and in my understanding it must be this way... and in my understanding I must not allow it to be devalued... this would devalue me, devalue my soul..." –Anonymous

This quote contains everything that we need to know about being human, humanity, and expression of the soul, yet our worldview turned it into a misunderstanding with wide-reaching consequences. We shortchanged this true love to one person in life. When everything is one and there is the same original divine energy in everything that exists, the above mentioned sentence would be as followed:

My deepest identity is the love of all that is... and this love is for me to protect, for otherwise I lose my identity, the meaning of life... to me, this is the greatest love on earth, and in my understanding it must be this way... and in my understanding I must not allow it to be devalued... this would devalue me, devalue my soul...

Being one with everything also means being aware – fully and unfiltered – of the pain of the environment. So far we have been unaware and, for this reason, we have subconsciously struck back, because we believed that the others out there are responsible. But when we are ever more aware of ourselves, we will recognize how these mechanisms operate, and an irresistible drive arises to change ourselves and the things around us that cause suffering. This drive grows incessantly, because it becomes clear that the entire existing worldview with its current systems oppose true peace, true health and true love. There is the wish to change the world, because we want to contribute to finally putting an end to the suffering and the illusion of separation.

By remembering this primordial part within us, we connect and confederate with each other regarding our oneness with precisely this primordial part in everything around us. Through this new understanding we uncover the misunderstandings and sources of our suffering.

With true self-confidence we are able to recognizes, that this "greatest love on earth" is the basic prerequisite for a MEANINGFUL life and ONENESS. Then, we possess the ADDED motivation that seemed so impossible. Then, we WANT to express who we truly are. Until now we believed that change is only possible in connection with severe suffering and force, and that we need to control people, while actually the exact opposite is true. The suffering and the ADDED are closely related anyway, but in an entirely different way. Previously it was an AWAY-FROM-MOTIVATION and SUFFERING, and now it can be an ADDED-MOTIVATION and ABSENCE OF SUFFERING, since love, joy, peace, health and abundance are allowed to appear in their place and we are content to control and lead ourselves. To achieve this, however, we must question everything that we have ever believed.

I am convinced that we as human beings are, figuratively speaking, in an early stage of development in terms of our true potential and possibilities and have created the world as it currently is out of our lack of understanding. We are, however, not in our baby or toddler shoes, but rather figuratively speaking in those of a schoolchild that exhibits dyslexia and dyscalculia. We are suffering symbolically from a misperception due to a developmental delay, that causes us to perceive numbers and letters both normally and mirror-inverted. This results in misinterpretations of things, people, feelings, numbers, data, facts and situations.

To clearly illustrate what I am referring to, I would like to include a few sample calculations of a child, that confuses right and left in its perception, and exhibits a different connection between the left and right brain.
For example, this child calculates:

   12 + 5 = 26 or 53 + 4 = 39
   36 + 2 = 83
   34 + 2 = 86

In closer examination we can see that this child also calculates properly, if we break away from our precast notion of the correct result. The child is calculating 1 + 5 = 6 and applying the 2 as a "ten number". In the second calculation, the same approach is applied, repeating this in other sample calculations. In the third sample, the child simply interchanged the numbers in the result. The last calculation, 34 + 2 = 86, is very interesting: here the child perceives the 3 in the number 34 as an 8. The 3 and the mirror image of the 3 are present simultaneously, which results in the image of an 8. At the same time, the child exhibits a misperception that has it interpret the letter F for example as the number 7; it sees the letter mirror-inverted. Thus we can realize, that this child also confuses numbers and letters, and sees them both normally and mirror-inverted. When you imagine the totality of possible false connections, both in reading and in calculations, it becomes clear how confusing perception must be and how difficult it is to produce a "correct" result. The results this child produces occur entirely logical in its world; they are merely logical in a different way, and wrong according to our standards. Learning to calculate and write poses a much greater challenge for such a child than for a normal child, at least until we discover exactly where and how this child perceives things differently.

It is much the same with our perception of oneness and separation, or of unconditional love and conditional love. We as humanity are like this child with its developmental delay and the resulting dyslexia and dyscalculia. We produce more than an average number of incorrect results, although we have fully comprehended the basic principles of success itself. Confusing left and right represent, figuratively speaking, the confusion of negative and positive. Just as the negative of a photograph makes it difficult to see what the original image looks like, and a specific, predefined development process is necessary so that we can see and register the actual image, we as human beings also require a developmental step. We do not recognize the "characters" properly and choose the "wrong" conclusions or combinations more often than usual in our currently limited and still delayed developmental stage.

The lack of this developmental process led previously to the confusion of numbers, data and facts, as well as feelings, that are calculated, read and combined using the logical calculation and reading connections that are inherent in all of us and represent true success, but with partial misinterpretations due to that confusion. Thus a worldview arises in which we somehow attempt to do the right thing, but nonetheless usually end up with the wrong result. How often we end up with a different result, than the one we should actually expect, but we don't know how we arrived there. Our success, our „heaven on earth", cannot be experienced – we have added things up incorrectly.

A Shift is possible in future, if we recognize that our way of living in this framework of developmental delay is not wrong, but should actually be seen as right in the context of our underlying conditions and our stage of development – in the sense that action causes reaction. There is, however, an overall frame of reference that forwards further development and improves and expands our perception significantly. When we recognize and acknowledge a new frame of reference, it is like we finally resolve this child's developmental deficit and its learning disabilities. Suddenly a new purpose is recognized and calculated, read and lived, and everything makes more and more sense. A correct result is attained. When internal and external truths are aligned with the universal laws of „mathematics and spelling", we can correctly combine any relationship – whether internal or external, tangible or intangible – and 1 + 1 finally equals 2. And, through the joy of finally resolving this developmental deficit, a potential growth of self-awareness, self-confidence, creativity, desire to grow, willingness to change and trust arises. We finally have the possibility to meaningfully apply the new capabilities in our daily life, to be understood and to understand others or even to help them; we finally belong and we do better at finding our way in life.

It is actually exponential growth – we can see this very clearly on an additional, very simple and everyday example. If we are designing a house and we modify the floor plan by one meter, we get exponential growth. We only add several centimeters to the blueprint, but in reality, one additional meter at a width of eight meters gives us eight square meters of additional floor space. What would be the consequences of such a small change in a PLAN? More time, material, financial means and room are needed for the planning, implementation, cleaning, maintenance and repairs; the appearance changes, etc. This in turn has an effect on every single person that is directly or indirectly involved in this project. For the people that are directly involved it can lead to additional stress. More money must be made, which means more work – on the job and for the cleaning and maintenance of the house – partners could grow apart, the children would no longer have quality time with their parents, and eventually the whole dream of home, sweet home has disappeared. Nobody reckoned with the whole string of events.

Countless things change subsequently when we change just this one parameter on a little blueprint. Herein lay the explanation of why we all too often master a challenge, only to create "ten new ones". As long as we are not aware that we are all connected to everything, we will continue to master one challenge – add one meter to our soul's house – without really considering all of the consequences, and create scads of new challenges. That is unless we are careful to ensure that changing is in alignment with the universal laws and the divine order.

With all of our differentiation, specification and separation, we have forgotten to be mindful of what unites - whether rich or poor, small or large, powerful or powerless, black or white, yellow or red, playful or serious, creative or boring, woman or man, adult or child – it is all about one thing: the HUMAN BEING in his/her totality, that carries all of these expressions somewhere within. If we continue on this path and also include the animal and plant kingdoms, as well as everything else that exists on this earth, we will then arrive at our origin. For all things have one thing in common: life – the divine universal energy and essence. Instead of separating we are called to unite again and, most importantly, to remember that beyond our sense of separation we have always been one. Together we can cause our light to shine; the light that has always been there.

Enlightenment

Enlightenment is to recognize ourselves in everything that surrounds us. It is claimed that Francis of Assisi was able to see beauty that others couldn't see. The reference here was not alone to the beauty in nature or everyday things, but rather the beauty in knowing and recognizing the divine universal presence, perfection and beauty in EVERYTHING that surrounds us – even those we dislike. It is the awareness of one's self and everything as it is truly intended, beyond any misunderstandings as we know them.
We live in duality, yet currently we do not act accordingly. Hot and cold, up and down, small and large allow us to recognize

and experience the complete scale of these conditions. We have forgotten, however, that as human beings, we can only experience things in duality, when we also acknowledge and experience the counterpart of our own divinity. Only then does being human truly make sense and only then we can live true humanity and enjoy our lives with all senses.

When more and more people recognize their light we can enlighten each other and together become an enlightened society, for we are aware that we are, have always been and always will be one with everything. Everything and everybody around us is our mirror, in which we recognize ourselves. Like playing „memory", everything inside of us has its „true other" out there, to recognize and remember who we truly are. While „searching" or more precisely waiting for the appearance of this „true other" counterpart in our perception, we experience our remembering and even recreation of ourselves and life itself. Oneness will then finally be experienced as a reflection of all desired and so-longed-for characteristics, and the negative reflections of our shadows and fears will gradually fade. The more people facilitate this positive reflection, the negative reflection will miss their „true other" but therefore the chance arise, that the now created positive counterpart will touch the misunderstood „true other" in those, who act out of their misunderstandings in an inaccurate way. The faster our lights are reflected, the faster people will realize and remember who they really are. We are all as mirror in our right position, but we have covered parts of our mirror, so that the light could not be reflected until now. We have always been ONE. Now it is just time to let all these covers and shadows go, so that we can reflect what is really out there, in order to become what we were longing for such a long time.

Enlightenment and true collective consciousness is the greatest pandemic of the world, and the snowball system the human misinterpretation is so deathly afraid of. It is the same fear it was, when man still believed the world was flat and then discovered that it isn't.

Internal and external wealth is possible, and basically has always been there – if we could BEGIN to REFRAIN from destroying the world and everything that lives, out of our misunderstanding of our divine origin and, with that, our strength and power. Together we could then create the world that we are all longing for. It can be created, if we stop doing what stands causally in opposition to love, our health and peace. The earth does not need to be saved, if we stop destroying its balance and self-healing. We have the opportunity to finally stop destroying ourselves, so that everything can be restored to the divine balance; to harmony with everything that exists.

The English words for remembering show us in profound truth what it is really all about:

RE-MIND: the word stem "re" means "again" or "back", while the word "mind" means intellect, understanding, "that, which reasons, thinks, feels, wills, perceives, judges, remembers", etc. This illustrates that this word means a general update, so to speak an actualization of our intellect, so that we can experience ourselves the UP-GRADE of our own higher-end configuration or vision of ourselves. Thinking, speaking, seeing, hearing, feeling and acting in alignment with the heart brings us the most all-encompassing recollection and understanding.

RE-MEMBER: we already discussed the word stem "re". The word "member" means part of a collective or body; a constituent part of any structural or composite whole. IT IS OUR DECISION, our free WILL, whether we chose to recognize ourselves as a member or part of the big picture, and to surrender to this. By exercising our free will here, we put ourselves in the position to experience oneness in the way we have always longed to. This oneness automatically leads to belonging and agreement, since this divine universal energy is apparent and recognizable in everything, thus we are all connected with the "one intelligence": the master spirit. Being in agreement is the logical consequence. This is our greatest upgrade so far, the truly greatest and best next version of ourselves.

ENLIGHTENMENT IS THE BIRTHRIGHT OF EACH HUMAN BEING and thus of ALL OF US, since we are ALL CONNECTED TO EVERYTHING AND THUS WERE ONE, ARE ONE AND REMAIN ONE. IT IS UP TO US WHETHER AND WHEN WE RECAPTURE OUR PARADISE AND OUR THRONE.

THANKS

I want to thank you for reading this book, and because I know that you will contribute in your own unique way to help create a better version of this world.

This book would not exist without the collaboration of many people and circumstances, and without their contributions you would never have been able to read it. This is why at this juncture I would like to give my deep, heartfelt thanks to everyone who came into my life as angels or "arsch- (ass-) angels, as Robert Betz likes to say. I also thank all those, who had to deal with my way of being an „ass-angel". I'm grateful that you all were so patient with me. I wished, I would have come to that point of my life without „hurting" so many people.
But together we helped to create this book, along with all those who never entered my life but though all manner of circumstances inspired me to think deeply about all these things.

I would like to express my very special thanks to my children, who were the source of many of my "why" questions. I knew right from the start that they had a gift for me, I just did not understand. It was always clear to me, however, that I would go through hell and back for my children if necessary which, figuratively speaking, I did in fact do. I love you, you three rascals and angels.

An especially big „thank you" also goes to my ex-husband Uwe, who continues to stand by my side in loving friendship, as I have by his, and has supported me in my most difficult times. How wonderful that you are here.

A deep gratitude goes to my parents; without whom I would never have been born. Beyond that, thanks to them I have had many experiences that contributed to making this book what it is.

Moreover, I want to give thanks to a very special man, a human being who came into my life as the soul mate, friend and mentor as described here in this book. He helped me change my life forever. I would never have had the idea to write a book, not to mention that I would never have had the courage to share it with the world. Thank you for being here.

I also want to thank my author coach, Gerhard Kilian, who gave me important pointers in the most important phase of the writing process, so that this book could turn out as it did. Our collaboration was great fun, highly instructive and very enriching. I'm really grateful that some coincidences lead me to my translator Herb Quick. He is really a multi-talented man with whom collaboration is a gift because he made the impossible thing possible. Thanks for being just you.

In addition, I wish to thank Robert Redford for his film The Legend of Bagger Vance, and Rachel Portman for her musical piece, Junuh Sees the Field. This film in general, and the music in particular, was repeatedly my re-connection and anchor to everything this book is about, and to heaven, which was finally within my grasp. The music was a key moment and a signpost on my path to the paradise within myself. This film has immeasurable depth and wisdom and is truly heaven-sent. Many thanks. Without the film, the music and phrases spoken exactly the way they were spoken, I would likely have misinterpreted the message of my heart, and this book would not have turned out the way it did. It was Bagger who said in the film, "Inside each and every one of us is one true authentic swing… somethin' we were born with… somethin' that's got to be remembered… Some folk even forget what their swing was like…" I believe that pretty much all people in this world have forgotten their own authentic swing of divine universal origin, and that it is all the more important now that we remember who we really are.

I want to thank Neale Donald Walsch, whose books were heart and eye-openers for me years ago already. His trilogy, Conversations with God, finally provided the answers I was never able to find in my church at the time and increased my range of awareness enormously. I truly believe your messages and therefore I lived them to experience what you can find in that book. Many thanks, Neale. In my darkest hours you were the one who showed me the way back to my life.

I also wish to thank Napoleon Hill for his book "Think and Grow Rich" which was a most enriching source of inspiration in various life situations and opened the doors to combine success and spirituality the way we did in this book.
There are countless more people whom I thank and are not mentioned here. You know who you are... I embrace you.

I thank the entire universe for guiding me to write this book, which continues to fills me with awe and amazement.

And I thank all of us for collectively making changes possible that serve us all. This is the greatest thanks that I could ever receive.

www.ingramcontent.com/pod-product-compliance
Lightning Source LLC
Chambersburg PA
CBHW070842160426
43192CB00012B/2274